# MIXED METHODS RESEARCH

# MIXED METHODS RESEARCH

MERGING THEORY WITH PRACTICE

Sharlene Nagy Hesse-Biber

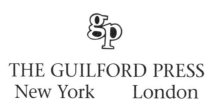

THE GUILFORD PRESS
New York      London

© 2010 The Guilford Press
A Division of Guilford Publications, Inc.
72 Spring Street, New York, NY 10012
www.guilford.com

Printed in the United States of America

This book is printed on acid-free paper.

Last digit is print number:   9   8   7   6   5   4   3   2   1

**Library of Congress Cataloging-in-Publication Data**

Hesse-Biber, Sharlene Nagy.
  Mixed methods research: merging theory with practice / Sharlene Nagy
Hesse-Biber.
    p. cm.
  Includes bibliographical references and index.
  ISBN 978-1-60623-259-0 (pbk.: alk. paper) — ISBN 978-1-60623-505-8 (hbk.:
alk. paper)
  1. Social sciences—Research—Methodology.   I. Title.
  H62.H477 2010
  001.4′2—dc22

                                                        2009044850

*To the incredibly gifted Boston, Massachusetts, medical doctors who continue to fight the battle against breast cancer each day—Patiksha Patel, Harold Burstein, Jay Harris, and Mehra Golshan. Thank you all so much for your expertise and support.*

# Preface

This book offers a comprehensive perspective on mixed methods research that emphasizes the central place of the *research problem* in mixed methods design and practice. The state of the field of mixed methods research is currently "methods-centric"; it focuses primarily on the construction of mixed methods designs, often to the detriment of how they interact with the research problem.

Lacking as well is an appreciation of the diversity of different methodological standpoints that currently employ a mixed methods approach or seek to do so. A plethora of mixed methods studies assume the standpoint of a positivist interpretation fueled by a growing movement in the social sciences toward more "evidence-based" research practice. Qualitative approaches to mixed methods remain marginalized in mainstream books and articles on the topic. If this point of view appears in a discussion of this method, it often takes on the standpoint of "second best." This book seeks to upend this relationship and perhaps turn it around in a variety of ways and to provide a reconceptualization of the mixed methods process through the lens of a qualitative approach.

Understanding the role and importance of mixed methods in social science research is a journey perhaps best taken together. This book makes use of the terms "we" and "our" in reference to the exploration that you, the reader, and I, the author, will conduct together throughout the course of this book. In doing so, we are consciously eliminating the traditional line that separates the authoritative voice of the author from the valuable input and experiences of the reader. In remaining open-minded about the relationship between author and reader, we hope to bridge the distance often imposed unnecessarily between them.

Continuing on the theme of dialogue within this book, we discuss how researchers taking a qualitative approach can successfully use mixed methods without having one component always taking on the "primary" role. We also discuss those specific research problems that particularly lend themselves to a mixed methods design, the process of generating a mixed methods question, and how to match a given research problem with a specific set of methods. I provide a set of reflexive strategies for finding your "research standpoint," and, in doing so, I hope this connection will serve to keep your research projects grounded and focused.

Along the way, we work through a set of suggested guidelines for generating a mixed methods research problem, dealing with specific ethical issues that may arise in conducting mixed methods research, as well as tips and procedures for gathering data, analyzing, interpreting, and writing up a mixed methods project.

We look at a set of in-depth case studies of mixed methods practice across a variety of qualitative approaches, starting with an overall discussion of the qualitative approach to mixed methods, as well as three specific approaches, with one chapter on interpretative research, another on qualitative feminist approaches, and the last on qualitative postmodern perspectives. I then take you through an extended example of the overall application of a qualitative mixed methods approach, breaking down the steps of putting together a mixed methods research design.

Along the way, I include "researcher standpoint" accounts from some leading scholars in the field of mixed methods research, asking them to personally and professionally reflect on their own experiences with mixed methods theory and practice. The work of some of these scholars and researchers is included among the in-depth case studies presented in this book.

Although the book centers on qualitative approaches to mixed methods research, it also provides space for dialogue among various researcher standpoints. I hope this book will be the beginning of a series of dialogues across methodological divides. The qualitative–quantitative methods divide is not the main issue confronting mixed methods research; rather, it is the absence of an awareness that all research comes from somewhere. In particular, this book is a call for researchers to grapple with and identify their particular standpoint on social reality and the construction of knowledge and to incorporate this awareness into their research practice at every stage, including, and most important, their choices about research methods and design. Some researchers may occupy multiple methodological standpoints, and these can shift and perhaps blend depending on, among other things, the particular research context, their methods training, and their acceptance of a diversity of theoretical perspectives. Researchers may find that they need to compromise or accommodate another's point of view as a project proceeds. It is nonetheless important that we are clear on what set of research standpoints we engage with in a research project.

There is a growing movement toward interdisciplinary research, and in the coming decades, this form of research structure will require a team-based approach, most likely working with researchers who occupy multiple research standpoints. There are often pressures on this kind of multidisciplinary research team to communicate across their methodological divides. In order for interdisciplinary work to be truly interdisciplinary, we must develop an awareness that knowledge building comes from a point of view, even if this may challenge more entrenched forms of knowledge building within a team. It may, in fact, come to pass that in the process of reaching over methodological divides, a renewed appreciation of the viewpoint(s) of the "other" will emerge, even if methodologies remain separate and divided within a project. Not all research projects should or need to mix their methodologies, but sometimes this process is important depending on the research goals of the project. In this case, methodological engagement can lead to a richer set of new questions ripe for mixed methods or emergent methods practice.

Let's begin our journey together....

# Acknowledgments

I would like to thank all those who have supported me along the way. First and foremost, I thank my family: my husband, neurologist and sleep specialist Michael Peter Biber, MD, whose love, sense of humor, and understanding is invaluable to me; and my daughters, Sarah Alexandra Biber, a Brandeis doctoral student majoring in genetics, and Julia Ariel Biber, City University of New York doctoral student majoring in cello performance, who support and cheer me on with my book projects but also remind me that there are other things in life besides writing a mixed methods book! I love you all!

My gratitude to my sister Georgia Gerraghty, my brother, Charles Nagy, and, of course, my mother, Helene Stockert, whose work ethic, guidance, and sound advice have inspired and sustained me throughout my academic and personal life.

A heartfelt remembrance of my sister Janet Mildred Nagy Green, whose life was cut short by breast cancer. Her wisdom, courage, humor, and love of life will always sustain me.

Very special thanks and my deepest gratitude go to several undergraduate research assistants and graduate students who have been instrumental to this project. I first want to give praise and thanks to Boston College graduate Natalie Horbachevsky, 2009, and undergraduate Alicia Johnson, 2011, for providing me with invaluable feedback and excellent editorial revisions on the book and for keeping things organized. My gratitude also to Boston College graduates Cooley Horner, 2009, and Lauren Kraics, 2009, and to Brandeis doctoral student Meg

Lovejoy, for their excellent research support and editorial work on this project.

I warmly acknowledge the contribution of Chris Kelly, doctoral student in the Sociology Department at Boston College, for his work as a contributor to the chapter on postmodernist approaches.

I also want to thank Boston College's undergraduate research grants office for their partial funding of this book project. My special thanks also to Dr. William Petri, Associate Dean, Arts and Sciences, Boston College, and the Boston College Undergraduate Research Fellowship Program. I would also like to thank the reviewers of the earlier drafts of the book, whose feedback was so helpful in shaping this book: Kai Schafft, Penn State University; Nancy Grudens-Schuck, Iowa State University; and Mark Earley, Bowling Green State University.

In addition, I offer my sincere thanks to C. Deborah Laughton, Publisher, Methodology and Statistics, at The Guilford Press. She is a gifted editor whose unwavering support, enthusiasm, expansive knowledge of the field of research methods, and outstanding editorial feedback on this book project is greatly appreciated. C. Deborah, you are one of a kind. Many thanks to Anna Nelson, Senior Production Editor at The Guilford Press, for her excellent editorial advice and finely honed skills that are so important in the final stages of the publishing process.

I want to thank and acknowledge a group of significant others within my community of friends and acquaintances who have in their own way supported me in this journey. I am grateful to Erin Kelly, my outstanding personal trainer, who makes my workouts challenging and fun. A warm thanks to my network of "early morning" people I meet up with at Peet's Coffee and who prefer to be called by their first names or nicknames: Ronnie, Mark, Jeff, Ellen, Bob, Toby, Larry, Jeffrey, Elaine, Rhonda, Sharon, and Jim. We are the "Peetniks," who hang out at our special table sipping coffee, enmeshed in thoughtful and humorous conversation, laughter, and sometimes tears.

# Contents

# CHAPTER 1

# Introduction to Mixed Methods Research

Mixed methods research designs are moving across the disciplines. Their influence is accelerating considerably, especially over the past decade. Researchers are witnessing an influx of mixed methods articles, books, and handbooks that tackle the thorny questions that challenge and push the boundaries of long-held foundational assumptions concerning how knowledge is built, what we can know, and how knowledge building ought to proceed.[1]

The growth of mixed methods research is a result of a convergence of factors. The influx of publications on mixed methods is certainly helping to boost its popularity. Additionally, external pressures to combine methods are coming from governmental and private funding agencies, evaluators, and other stakeholders who increasingly want researchers to utilize mixed methods to explore social policy issues.

The advent of new computer-based technologies is sparking great interest in combining a variety of new mixed methods designs and analytical practices. Computer-assisted qualitative data analysis software programs (CAQDAS), for example, have the ability to incorporate quantitative data into their programs. Qualitative researchers are now able to create quantitative measures from their qualitative data, a statistical measure that was not available for use until recently (Hesse Bibcr & Leavy, 2006b; Sandelowski, Volis, & Knafl, 2009).

There is also a growing demand for methods that address the range and scope of novel research questions emanating from new theoretical contributions. The pioneering works of feminists, postcolonialists, postmodernists, and critical theorists aims to expose subjugated knowledge of oppressed groups that has often been left out of or ignored in traditional research. These new paradigms look at the intersections of race, class, gender, nationality, and other hierarchical forms of social identity and often pinpoint subjugated groups as the focus of social inquiry. Feminist standpoint theory (Harding, 2004; Smith, 1987b), for example, places women's concerns, knowledge, and experiences at the forefront of academic concern and inquiry and is committed to issues of social justice and societal change for women. Critical theory and critical race theory (Wing, 2000) contest traditional knowledge forms and expose the power dynamics of traditional knowledge by revealing the interactions among gender, race, class, nationality, and other social identities. Mixed methods research holds greater potential to address these complex questions by acknowledging the dynamic interconnections that traditional research methods have not adequately addressed (Hesse-Biber & Crofts, 2008; Hesse-Biber & Leavy, 2006b).

Mixed methods research developed with the earliest social research projects; among these are studies of poverty within families conducted in the 1800s in Europe by researchers such as Frédéric Le Play (1855), Charles Booth (1892–1897), and Bohm Rowntree (1901). Their research practices include the incorporation of quantitative and qualitative techniques, including the use of demographic analysis, participant surveys and observations, and social mapping techniques. Charles Booth, for example, developed a social cartography of the city of London by color-coding streets by social class and income of their population. These emergent methods practices filtered into the research landscape in the United States by the beginning of the 20th century (Gilgun, 1999). The Chicago School of Sociology, founded in the 1920s, is noted for its prominence in urban ethnography with an emphasis on a qualitative "case study" approach. The founders of the Chicago School also employed quantitative data (Bulmer, 1984, p. 6). Robert Park, a core member of the Chicago School, applied a mixed methods approach to the study of inner-city urban life by integrating both qualitative and quantitative data into his case studies. He found quantitative data particularly valuable as a marker of social processes. Martin Bulmer (1984) noted:

> Park's main emphasis in urban theory was upon processes of invasion and succession and the natural histories of groups and areas

within the city. He wrote in 1926: "In so far as social structure can be defined in terms of position, social changes may be defined in terms of movement: and society exhibits in one of its aspects that can be measured and described in mathematical formulas." He took an interest in land values, or street-car transfers, or the volume of traffic at intersections, as indexes for underlying social processes. (p. 153)

## What Are Mixed Methods?

In general, researchers who use mixed methods employ a research design that uses both quantitative and qualitative data to answer a particular question or set of questions. This combination of methods "involve[s] the collection, analysis, and integration of quantitative and qualitative data in a single or multiphase study" (Hanson, Creswell, Plano Clark, Petska, & Creswell, 2005, p. 224). The term "multimethods" refers to the mixing of methods by combining two or more qualitative methods in a single research study (such as in-depth interviewing and participant observation) or by using two or more quantitative methods (such as a survey and experiment) in a single research study.

Mixed methods is a rich field for the combination of data because with this design "words, pictures, and narrative can be used to add meaning to numbers" (Johnson & Onwuegbuzie, 2004, p. 21). In other words, what we generally consider qualitative data—"words, pictures, and narrative"—can be combined with quantitative, numerical data from a larger-scale study on the same issue, allowing our research results to be generalized for future studies and examinations.

## Why Use Mixed Methods?

Greene, Caracelli, and Graham (1989) list five specific reasons that researchers should consider using mixed methods. The first, *triangulation*, seems to be the most commonly cited reason that mixed methods are incorporated into research. Triangulation—or, more specifically, *methods triangulation*, in the context of methods alone—refers to the use of more than one method while studying the same research question in order to "examine the same dimension of a research problem" (Jick, 1979, p. 602). The researcher is looking for a convergence of the data collected by all methods in a study to enhance the credibility of the research findings. Triangulation ultimately fortifies and enriches a study's conclusions, making them more acceptable to advocates of both qualitative and quantitative methods.

The second reason to consider incorporating a mixed methods design is *complementarity*. Complementarity allows the researcher to gain a fuller understanding of the research problem and/or to clarify a given research result. This is accomplished by utilizing both quantitative and qualitative data and not just the numerical or narrative explanation alone to understand the social story in its entirety. Both complementarity and triangulation are useful "for cross-validation when multiple methods produce comparable data" (Yauch & Steudel, 2003, p. 466). Complementarity has proven useful in several research studies, and a strong example is Yauch and Steudel's (2003) examination of the organizational cultures of two small manufacturers. In their work, Yauch and Steudel utilized both qualitative and quantitative research methods. Not only did the triangulation of the qualitative and quantitative data secure the validity of their study, but the complementarity of the two datasets produced a more thorough comprehension of the organizational cultures in question.

The researchers first used employee interviews to gather a wealth of narrative information and then used their qualitative findings to create a survey to collect numerical data. Yauch and Steudel's hope was to use mixed methods to "identify key cultural factors that aided or hindered a company's ability to successfully implement manufacturing cells [autonomous labor teams]" (2003, p. 467). Combining and crossing these data yielded rich results:

> Despite the long delay between beginning the qualitative assessment and administering the survey, the OCI [survey] was an important means of triangulation for two of the cultural factors identified and had the potential to reveal additional cultural dimensions that the qualitative analysis might have missed. (Yauch & Steudel, 2003, p. 476)

This study illustrates the power and possibilities inherent in mixed methods research; the researchers unearthed the convergence of the data from interviews and surveys through triangulation as well as the complementarity of the qualitative and quantitative data, which supplied them with a greater understanding of the organizational cultures of small manufacturers.

Mixed methods assist the researcher's total understanding of the research problem; this understanding represents the third reason for using mixed methods: *development*. Mixed methods often aid in the development of a research project by creating a synergistic effect, whereby the "results from one method . . . help develop or inform the other method" (Greene et al., 1989, p. 259). For example, statistical data collected from a quantitative method can often shape interview questions for the qualitative portion of one's study. Jenkins's (2001) research on rural adolescents and substance abuse illustrates the potential of the development factor in a mixed methods study. Jenkins administered a structured questionnaire to quantitatively measure students' drug use. Her study also included a follow-up set of focus-group interviews and open-ended questionnaires intended to capture students' perceptions of "drug resistance difficulties" to a variety drugs ranging from alcohol to LSD to various types of narcotics (Jenkins, 2001, p. 215). The results from conducting both these studies sequentially contributed to Jenkins's overall understanding of drug abuse among this population. Her initial use of a structured questionnaire provided her with a statistical understanding of student drug use. A follow-up focus-group study provided her the opportunity to triangulate her data (asking whether the findings from both studies agreed), and, in doing so, she found that the results from the focus group were "consistent with the open-ended questionnaire findings . . . [and] provided further clarification and, in some instances, additional information" (Jenkins, 2001, p. 219). In addition, by implementing a sequential design with the quantitative component first and the qualitative second, she was able to attain a "value added" understanding of the results from both studies. Her focus-group data allowed her to clarify and follow up on definitions and uses of terms, such as "peer pressure," that were used in survey questions and to ground their meaning from the perspective of her respondents.

A fourth reason cited for using mixed methods is *initiation*; a study's findings may raise questions or contradictions that will require clarification, thus initiating a new study. The desired effect of the new study would be to add new insights to existing theories on the phenomenon under examination (Greene et al., 1989). In fact, findings from this study might uncover a completely new social research topic and launch a new investigation, leading us to a fifth reason for doing mixed methods research: *expansion*. Expansion is intended to "extend the breadth and range of the inquiry" (Greene et al., 1989, p. 259). Producing detailed findings helps enable future research endeavors and allows researchers to continuously employ different and mixed methods in their pursuit of new or modified research questions.

Greene and her colleagues (1989) provide a useful organizing framework for characterizing the ways researchers have used mixed methods. We can clearly see the positive power and synergy of using these methods to complement one's research findings. Quantitative information delivered in a "hard data" format is amenable to statistical analyses and standardized tests of reliability and validity. Qualitative data add an in-depth understanding of research results and allow the researcher to explore anomalies or subgroups within the data. Working with both methods gives many researchers a cross-check on their research results. Qualitative data illuminate the meaning of statistical results by adding a narrative understanding to quantitative research findings. Qualitative methods can also assist researchers who want to test the validity of their research questionnaires by sequentially utilizing mixed methods. For instance, an initial qualitative study allows the development of research instruments, such as a questionnaire, that can be used in a large-scale quantitative research study. Similarly, quantitative data can assist qualitative researchers by providing them with a broader context within which to place their qualitative data, as well as providing, through survey samples, ways to identify representative cases for their in-depth research. It is in this sense that quantitative data can be useful for establishing generalizability of qualitative results.

All of these reasons provide strong arguments for a researcher to consider a mixed methods approach. The following in-depth example shows the promise of mixed methods research in tackling a complex social problem: obesity in children.

### The Fight against Childhood Obesity:
### An Illustration of the Need for and Importance of Mixed Methods

America is facing a new range of problems in the 21st century. Poverty, war, and health care are among these challenges, but a deeper problem threatens families and children across the country. Childhood obesity has become a nationwide epidemic, and parents and physicians alike are raising concerns. Consider the following article that appeared in *The New York Times*:

> Six-year-old Karlind Dunbar barely touched her dinner, but not for time-honored 6-year-old reasons. The pasta was not the wrong shape. She did not have an urgent date with her dolls.
>
> The problem was the letter Karlind discovered, tucked inside her report card, saying that she had a body mass index in the 80th

percentile. The first grader did not know what "index" or "percentile" meant, or that children scoring in the 5th through 85th percentiles are considered normal, while those scoring higher are at risk of being or already overweight.

Yet she became convinced that her teachers were chastising her for overeating.

Since the letter arrived, "my 2-year-old eats more than she does," said Georgeanna Dunbar, Karlind's mother, who complained to the school and is trying to help her confused child. "She's afraid she's going to get in trouble," Ms. Dunbar said. (Kantor, 2007, pp. A1, A14)[2]

Many school districts across the country have adopted the body mass index (BMI) screening test as a weapon for fighting childhood obesity. On the surface, conducting BMI screening tests on students from kindergarten through eighth grade appears to achieve an important health goal by identifying the percentage of children who are overweight, a crucial step in fighting childhood obesity. Yet there does not seem to be a research design in place that can fully address this objective if the goal of these data is to assist in stemming the tide of obesity. In fact, it appears as though little thought was ever given as to how these data might empower parents and their children to be part of the problem's solution. Gathering descriptive quantitative data is not enough to complete the goals of this study. One needs a broader understanding of the social context within which this information is disseminated among families to ensure that both students and parents are prepared to prevent childhood obesity and to develop the best strategy for fighting the obesity epidemic now.

There are many questions we might ask to gain a clearer understanding of the factors nurturing America's obesity problem. Exploring the lived experiences of students and their families and the day to-day experiences of children's eating behaviors at school would provide beneficial information. What is the school environment like for students with respect to eating? What types of relationships do they have with food at home? To what extent, if any, would parents welcome the school's input into their children's issues with weight? These are only a few of the many social-context questions that should be addressed so that schools might utilize the best approach for conveying weight-related "bad news" to both students and their families.

Designing a stronger research strategy would play a significant role in this process. For example, one might use a qualitative focus-group-study design following the collection of BMI scores. The quantitative data collected could be presented to a representative group of parents; the researchers, perhaps in conjunction with school and health officials, could assess the parents' reactions to this aggregated data for their school and also receive input on how to disseminate, if at all, these results to families and students. A mixed methods study consisting of a quantitative component (the BMI score collection) followed by a qualitative component (focus group) might give researchers a deeper understanding of parents' feelings and attitudes toward childhood obesity. The focus group could also collect parents' suggestions as to how these results could be utilized to combat the epidemic. As one mother quoted in *The New York Times* article commented, "The school provides us with this information with no education about how to use it or what it means" (Kantor, 2007, p. A14). A fictitious causal link exists in many researchers' minds that letters to parents will trigger the logical response of parents taking personal action to stem the tide of weight gain in their children. This strategy has not succeeded, and, in some cases, the opposite reaction seems to have occurred. One report observed the reaction of some parents: "the letters sent home with report cards . . . [were] a shock. Many parents threw them out, outraged to be told how much their children should weigh or unconvinced that children who look just fine by local standards are too large by official ones" (Kantor, 2007, p. A14).

In the end, rather than fighting the effects of obesity, the letter made many families feel helpless and victimized by a flawed system. There appears to be little understanding of the physical and mental effects of bad BMI news on parents and children. The assumption that the problem stems from imprinted eating habits learned at home leads to the conclusion that BMI screenings conducted in school would be an effective deterrent to childhood obesity. Yet research has revealed that the problem runs deeper than family eating habits and screenings. In some schools, the food available in the cafeterias was not nutritious and, in fact, exacerbated the problem. In these specific schools, cafeteria cuisine was the central root of the problem, as schools were "continuing to feed them atrocious quality meals and snacks, with limited if any opportunities for phys-ed in school" (Kantor, 2007, p. A14).

This example illustrates the need for mixed methods research across a range of disciplines from the physical sciences to the social and behavioral sciences. The problems that followed the BMI screening tests and information letters could have been assuaged with a unique research method that would probe the numerical and statistical data and unite it with qualitative information collected through interviews with parents and students so that an effective means of childhood obesity prevention and reversal might be discovered. Scholars and researchers are still debating the benefits of mixing methods, but there seems to be significant promise for this revolutionary design.

## Objectives of This Book

One objective of this book is to reconceptualize the approach to mixed methods research by offering a *comprehensive approach* that stresses the *tight link between theory and research* and that centers the research problem in the design and analysis of mixed methods projects, whether they are derived from a quantitative or a qualitative approach.

A second aim of this book is to center *qualitative approaches* to mixed methods research. Typically, in mixed methods research discourse, quantitative approaches have primacy over qualitative ones. Qualitative approaches stem from a different research logic, one that privileges subjective experience and that is open to a multilayered view of the social world. In this book, we focus on the idea that centering a qualitative approach in mixed methods research can be illuminating, useful, and advantageous, especially as a means to get at subjugated knowledge— knowledge that has not been a part of mainstream research inquiry. A mixed methods approach also allows the researcher to get at "subjective experiences" of those researched while providing the means to test out theories generated from in-depth research samples.

A third objective is to provide researchers with a more detailed understanding of qualitative mixed methods perspectives and practices. In addition, it is my hope that those researchers currently practicing mixed methods from a quantitative approach may dialogue with qualitative approaches by reflecting on the ways in which they might integrate a qualitative perspective into their mixed methods practice.

A final goal for this book is visionary and elusive. It is my wish that, in uncovering and centering qualitative approaches to mixed methods, we can open up a dialogue across current mixed methods research approaches and practices that may serve to fuel synergy and innovation in methods practice with the goal of providing a more complex view and understanding of the social world.

# A Comprehensive Perspective on Mixed Methods

I argue that the current practice of mixed methods research is exemplified by a "cart before the horse" approach. Mixed methods designs are driven by research techniques to the detriment of theory-based research. Figure 1.1 presents a "methods-centric" approach to mixed methods research that places methodology (theory) last in the process of choosing a particular mixed methods design. In this mixed methods design (Figure 1.1), methodology (theory) is isolated from the rest of the research model and appears as the last in the design sequence. It is not clear how theory (whether it is implied or explicit) is linked to a specific methods design, but it appears as if the mixed methods design model *is methods-centric* in that the type of mixed method model selected drives the type of theory chosen.

In their review of trends and issues in mixed methods evaluation, Miller and Fredericks (2006) suggested that this misplacement of theory in a mixed methods project is a "problem of logic" that often plagues the choice of mixed methods approaches, especially in evaluation research. They noted:

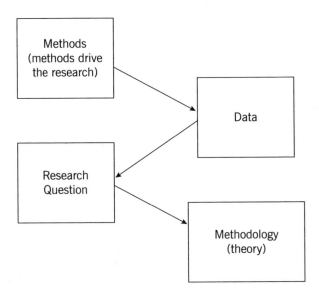

**FIGURE 1.1.** Methods-centric approach to mixed methods research.

One can, of course, a priori, simply declare that any MM strategy is appropriate for the issue being studied. However, this thinking introduces an unwanted arbitrariness to the whole process, which potentially undermines the very purpose of advocating for the uniqueness of MM. The situation is further exacerbated by the use of vague rationales for the selection of a particular mixed method, suggesting that the use of MM will result in richer data or stronger inferences. (p. 569)

As I have stated, I believe that current practice of mixed methods research takes a "cart before the horse" approach. I propose, instead, a practice of mixed methods that is firmly rooted within a research context with the intention that the method or methods used foster a richer understanding of the research problem under investigation.

## A Comprehensive Approach to Mixed Methods

Figure 1.2 provides a diagram of a comprehensive approach to research. The basic premise of the comprehensive approach is that methodology provides the theoretical perspective that links a research problem with a particular method or methods. Methodologies are derived from a researcher's assumptions about the nature of existence (ontology). These assumptions, in turn, lead to their perspective philosophy or set of philosophies on the nature of knowledge building (epistemology) regarding such foundational questions as: Who can know? What can be known? We can think of methodology as a theoretical bridge that connects the research problem with the research method. Kushner (2002) underscored the importance of methodology in methods practice:

> We cannot talk of "method" alone. To talk about the "interview" apart from its purpose is merely to picture two people engaged in verbal exchange. Only when we shift to the level of methodology where we talk about purpose and value does the instrument become sufficiently complex to sustain discussion. Method is like a glove which needs the human hand to give it shape and meaning. (p. 252)

Methodology leads the researcher to ask certain research questions and prioritize what questions and issues are most important to study. Researchers within and across disciplines can hold a range of different methodologies that frame their methods practice. They might

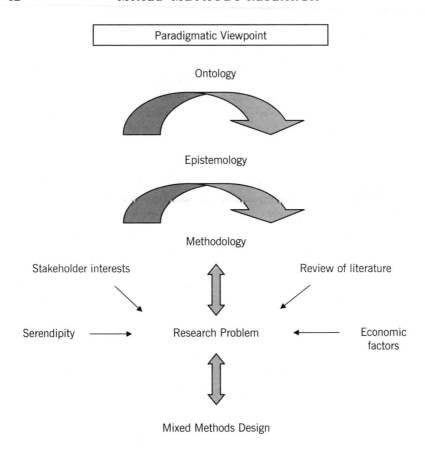

**FIGURE 1.2.** Comprehensive approach to mixed methods research.

use methodologies that hold up the importance of studying the "lived experiences" of individuals (interpretative methodologies), those that privilege hypothesis testing and causality as the most important goals of social inquiry (positivist and postpositivist methodologies), or methodologies that stress issues of power, control, and social justice (transformative and critical methodologies).

A methodological perspective is not inherently quantitative or qualitative in terms of its use of method. For example, those who practice more positivistic methodology—traditionally seen as quantitative—can use qualitative as well as quantitative methods. In fact, qualitative and quantitative methods are carried out within a range of methodologies (theoretical perspectives). Those espousing feminist methodologies—traditionally viewed as qualitative researchers—can use quantitative methods, including surveys and experiments, in their research. The comprehensive perspective on mixed methods troubles the dualism between qualitative and quantitative methods when we remember that methods lie in the service of methodologies.

Jennifer Greene (2002) captured the important role that a methodological framework takes on in a research project:

> Most . . . methodologies have preferences for particular methods, but methods gain meaning only from the methodologies that shape and guide their use. . . . An interview does not inherently respect the agency of individual human life; it only does so if guided by and implemented within a methodological framework that advances this stance. So, any discussions of mixing methods . . . must be discussions of mixing methodologies, and thus of the complex epistemological and value-based issues that such an idea invokes. (p. 260)

Greene stated that methods are tools and that, in the hands of researchers with certain methodological persuasions, they can be used to promote social justice, maintain the status quo, or promote social transformation. There is a need, then, for researchers to be conscious of the methodological perspective(s) they employ within their research projects. Greene, Benjamin, and Goodyear (2001) referred to this as "thoughtful mixed method planning," in which the researcher is cognizant of his or her particular methodological standpoint. They noted that each researcher should "figure out one's stance on the 'paradigm issues' in mixed method enquiry" (pp. 29–30). Good mixed methods work requires "consciousness of this organizing framework and adherence to its guidance for enquiry practice" (p. 30).

It is also important to note, however, that although paradigmatic assumptions very often guide the researcher in a variety of ways—including the selection of certain research problems, the choice of methods selected, and how the researcher will analyze and interpret his or her data—research questions can be guided by a range of additional factors. Figure 1.2 depicts these factors as arrows that can influence the research question. Influential factors can include a review of the research literature, specific constraints the researcher is faced with (both economic and lifestyle choices, as well as those particular constraints imposed by funding agencies and/or one's disciplinary practice), and even serendipity; these factors can preclude or favor the choice of particular research problems.

Sometimes a researcher is conscious about his or her paradigmatic worldview, but it can also remain implicit or even unconscious and taken for granted. Although there may be additional factors (economic concerns, time constraints, stakeholder interests) to take into account in the selection of a research method, methodology (theoretical perspective) is the link that connects the research question with specific methods that address these questions (see Jackson, 2006). We take up these issues in depth in Chapter 2.

## The Need for Qualitative Approaches to Mixed Methods Research

The mixed methods research design that appears to be the favored design model incorporates a qualitative component into a primarily quantitative study, as this model is thought to satisfy the need for generalization and to provide the illustrative power of narrative (Morse, 2003). This is not to discount the fact that there are mixed methods designs in which the qualitative component is primary, but even within these mixed methods studies, the goal of the qualitative component is often to "assist" the quantitative data in developing, for example, better measures for a survey or to assist in teasing out contradictory survey findings (Creswell, Shope, Plano Clark, & Green, 2006).

This popular type of mixed methods model is based on a quantitative *positivistic approach* to mixed methods research, one that privileges the scientific method of knowledge building. This type of science is built on a primarily deductive mode of knowledge building that relies on "theory testing" and that privileges value neutrality and objectivity over subjectively derived knowledge. Positivism holds the central belief that an objective reality exists that is independent of any individual's subjective experience. Quantitative data and analyses (using surveys, experiments, and statistical analysis of data) are often at the center, with qualitative data used in the service of enhancing a primarily quantitative mixed methods approach. Creswell, Plano Clark, Gutmann, and Hanson (2003) note that one of the most common mixed methods designs is triangulation (QUAN + QUAL). This design is employed when a researcher seeks to validate quantitative statistical findings with qualitative data results. Yet the assumption underlying triangulation is the positivistic view that there is an objective reality in which a given truth can be validated. The most common type of sequential mixed methods design appears to place the qualitative study in a more supportive role, "where qualitative pilot work is likely to precede and be subservient to a larger survey" (Brannen, 2005, p. 15). Bahl and Milne

(2006) note that within marketing research most researchers employ a "positivist orientation," using qualitative research in a "supportive role" to a more privileged quantitative study (p. 198).

Giddings (2006) noted the extent to which much of the mixed methods research has been conducted under the guise of a positivistic methodology—what she called, "positivism dressed in drag":

> A design is set in place, a protocol followed. In the main, the questions are descriptive, traditional positivist research language is used with a dusting of words from other paradigms, and the designs come up with structured descriptive results. Integration is at a descriptive level. A qualitative aspect of the study is often "fitted in." The thinking is clearly positivist and pragmatic. The message often received by a naïve researcher, however, is that mixed methods combines and shares "thinking" at the paradigm level. (p. 200)

According to Giddings, the idea that mixed methods research now combines the best of both qualitative and quantitative approaches is like a "new guise" for positivism and is really business as usual (2006, p. 200). In a sense, Giddings argued that mixed methods would serve only to strengthen the positivistic paradigm if in fact qualitative approaches were just "added and stirred" into a general positivistic methodological approach (p. 202). Although mixed methods approaches are not necessarily problematic in and of themselves, the consistent privileging of a quantitative approach in mixed methods research threatens to obscure the power and utility of qualitative approaches and the contributions they can make to mixed methods research.

There are few studies that analyze how mixed methods researchers are in fact using mixed methods designs in a range of empirical articles across the disciplines. What research exists suggests that researchers primarily use mixed methods at the "data collection" stage of a mixed methods project. Bryman (2006), in a content analysis of mixed methods articles, notes that for the most part the quantitative and qualitative portions of the studies were not integrated. In interviews with mixed methods researchers, Bryman (2007a) noted several reasons given by researchers for nonintegration. An important reason was the set of methodological biases researchers had toward one type of methodological approach. Researchers also mentioned the issue of the lag time between the two studies, especially with regard to the qualitative component of a study. Researchers also expressed confusion as to actually how to mix methods, especially at the data analysis and interpretation stages of a mixed methods project.

One missing piece in the discussion of mixed methods as a research design is the absence of its negative impact. We might critically ask questions such as, When is applying more methods detrimental or unnecessary to answering a given question? What are the economic costs of an additional methods component? What set of criteria helps the researcher decide when one method will do? What are the unintended consequences of applying a mixed methods design for the analysis and interpretation of data from both studies when the researcher is not adequately skilled in the application of both methods? These are but a few caveats regarding the employment of a mixed methods research design; what is more troublesome is that much of the mixed methods literature does not discuss the disadvantages of utilizing a mixed methods design.

This book's focus is on qualitative approaches, both mature and cutting edge, that enhance our understanding of the social world, particularly the lived experiences of individuals and groups. A focus on qualitative approaches to mixed methods research also fits well with the movement toward *interdisciplinary scholarship* that is placing pressure on researchers to draw from many disciplinary methodologies and traditions. Focusing on a range of qualitative approaches can provide a broader theoretical lens through which to look at novel and often thorny interdisciplinary research problems and issues. Qualitative approaches also allow researchers to incorporate issues of *social change, power,* and *authority* that push on the boundaries of traditional positivist and postpositivist research concerns and challenge what constitutes "legitimate" research.

Qualitative methodological approaches stress the importance of multiple subjective realities as an important source of knowledge building. Epistemology in this paradigm holds that knowledge gathering and truth are always partial; that researcher values, feelings, and attitudes cannot be removed from the research relationship but instead should be taken into consideration when interpreting the data as part of the knowledge construction process; and some of these approaches also argue that the researcher should establish a reciprocal relationship with research participants to promote an interactional, cooperative co-construction of meaning.

In this book, I demonstrate both the strength of qualitative methodologies and how, when, and why these approaches may best be combined with quantitative methods in mixed method designs. This perspective is developed and illustrated throughout the book with in-depth examples of how researchers with a qualitative approach employ mixed methods designs.

Researchers originally trained in positivist approaches to research may want to explore the extent to which qualitative methods and methodologies can assist them in answering their research questions. Qualitative approaches to research questions can be valuable to posi-tivistic researchers in a variety of ways, from assisting with the genera-tion of theories and models to the testing of these models. Qualitative approaches, with their emphasis on participant meaning and experi-ence, can also provide a much-needed context for the development of a range of survey instruments from assessment and evaluation tools to question items on surveys.

Qualitative methodologies are a particularly sensitive means of capturing the lived experiences of groups and individuals, especially those often left out of traditional knowledge-building research proj-ects. In other words, qualitative approaches such as postmodernism and feminist critical theory desire to explore the subjective worlds of multiple realities, uncover perspectives of those who have been socially and politically marginalized, and upend positivism's claims to objectiv-ity and traditional knowledge building as the source of truth.

Qualitative methodologies should not be mistaken for qualitative methods. Qualitative methodologies, as noted earlier, use quantitative as well as qualitative methods. The same rule applies for quantitative methodologies. After all, the method is but the tool; the methodology determines the way in which the tool will be utilized. This makes the issue of which design to use confusing and problematic for researchers working from a qualitative or quantitative methodological perspective. Early on, Lincoln and Guba (1985) noted that "naturalistic inquiry" was not necessarily antipositivistic and that, although the use of qualita-tive data allow the experiences of respondents to be voiced within the research project, there may be many ways in which quantitative data can be incorporated into this type of research approach (pp. 198–199).

This book highlights the ways in which a qualitative approach informs how mixed methods research is conducted. Not all qualitative approaches are the same, and I use this term as an umbrella category that encompasses several different approaches that have slightly differ-ent emphases. This book selects three specific qualitative approaches—an interpretative approach, a feminist approach, and a postmodern approach—to provide a more specific application of a qualitative approach to mixed methods research designs.

For each approach (the interpretative, feminist, and postmodern-ist approaches), we are interested in how researchers with these spe-cific qualitative points of view integrate mixed methods into their work. How conscious or unconscious is the process of choosing to utilize mixed methods? More specifically, what motivations or purposes can be discerned as reasons for mixing methods? In what way(s), if any, are the qualitative and quantitative components of a project related, and at what stage in the research process? What are the issues and positive outcomes of using a mixed methods design?

Each of these approaches to research makes certain ontologi-cal, epistemological, and methodological assumptions regarding the nature of the social world. These different theoretical approaches are often subsumed under the term "qualitative methodologies." However, these methodologies are just as diverse as the researchers who practice them, so let's take a moment to examine these different perspectives in greater depth.

If a researcher employs an *interpretative approach* to research, the researcher's epistemology assumes multiple subjective realities that consist of stories or meanings produced or constructed by individuals within their "natural" settings. Crabtree and Miller (1999) noted that interpretivists in particular

> trace their roots back to phenomenology (Schutz, 1967) and herme-neutics (Heidegger, 1927, 1962). This tradition also recognizes the importance of the subjective human creation of meaning but doesn't reject outright some notion of objectivity. Pluralism, not relativism, is stressed, with focus on the circular dynamic tension of subject and object. (p. 10)

*Feminist perspectives* are specifically interested in understanding knowledge "for women." These perspectives, such as standpoint theory, are aware of the "male-centered" biases of traditional positivistic con-cerns, especially as they pertain to the issues of objectivity within the research process whereby individuals must place their own values and concerns outside the research endeavor. For feminist researchers, there is no knowledge that is without bias. There is no view from "nowhere"; knowledge is imbued with the power and authority of those who have it. They point to the long-standing androcentric (male) bias of early knowledge building, especially as practiced by early positivists, which often ignored women's concerns in their research. Positivist research-ers have also historically overlooked issues of difference in terms of race, class, ethnicity, and sexual preference in their research problems and analyses, issues of difference that often centrally inform the work of feminist researchers. A *feminist perspective* moves the issues of those whose lives have been marginalized, overlooked, or misrepresented by traditional investigations to the "front and center" of the research agenda (see Hesse-Biber, 2007). Feminist research stresses the importance of intersectionality—standpoints or worldviews created by the overlapping of a combination of locations within the social structure (i.e., race, class, gender, sexuality, geography, etc.).

*Postmodern* theorists stress a relativistic approach in their treatment of the social construction of reality. Postmodernism—as well as its related schools of thought, poststructuralism and critical theory—emerged in the late 20th century with the goal of challenging the status quo of modern enlightenment thought. One defining feature of postmodernist paradigms is that they assume that images, symbols, texts, and other representations have the power to create and sustain a given social reality. We use "postmodernism" as an umbrella term for these theories; however, that does not mean that they are the same thing, and at times these terms may not be internally consistent with one another.

Postmodernism challenges positivism's emphasis on objective truth and instead posits how dominant discourse/language serves to oppress and maintain existing power relations within a society. Postmodernism focuses on deconstructing dominant images, symbols, and texts in order to disrupt their meanings and question their veracity, often by pointing out their class, race, and gender biases. Postmodernism favors a multilayered understanding of social reality that some critics of this perspective say borders on a relativistic view of the social world that obviates all of the scientific methods' claims to truth.

## Qualitative Mixed Methods Approaches: Some Examples

In this section, I provide two examples of researchers who employ a qualitative approach to mixed methods and highlight the ways in which their specific researcher standpoints serve to guide their decision making at various stages throughout the research process.

### A Feminist Approach

A feminist approach to knowledge building seeks to ask a set of research questions that often upend traditional forms of knowledge building by privileging the lived experiences of women at the center of research inquiry (feminist standpoint theory). Their theoretical perspective influences the type of research questions and the specific methods chosen, including the application of these methods in the data collection, analysis, and interpretation stages of the research process. A feminist methodology is firmly rooted in a specific theoretical standpoint on the nature of existence (ontology) and what can be known about it (epistemology). A feminist perspective does influence one's methods practice. For example, feminist researchers are particularly interested in issues of power, authority, and control while conducting research, and therefore they specifically explore such questions as: What is studied and why? From whose perspective is it studied? Who is studied? Who is left out and needs to be included in this study? Looking at difference is an integral part of their research agenda. Realizing that not all women are the same, there is a particular interest in how race, class, sexual orientation, and other differences intersect to impact specific women's lives.

Feminist researchers utilize a range of both quantitative and qualitative tools to answer research questions and are not wedded to one specific method or set of methods. They use whatever methods will best answer the research problem. The practice of research methods is mindful of the ways in which power and authority influence the research process.

### Applying Mixed Methods: Behind the Scenes with David A. Karp

David A. Karp is a qualitative researcher who has done cutting-edge research on mental illness. He brings a symbolic interaction with the social world and a theoretical perspective that focuses on how people experience, define, and make meaning out of their daily worlds. He is particularly interested in the experiences of those individuals who are suffering from depression and other mental illnesses. I conducted a set of intensive interviews with him for a behind-the-scenes glimpse into how researchers talk about conducting their own research and the struggles they face in doing so. He highlights the importance of placing methodology first in our understanding of the research process. He demonstrates how it is the researcher's theoretical perspective that leads her or him to ask certain questions, supporting the idea that the methodology of a researcher must be considered prior to deciding which methods to employ in order to acquire their answers.

In his research on depression, David Karp wants to understand depression on a micro rather than a macro level. His questions do not aim at the larger picture of depression—the numbers of people affected by this illness, the economic impact of the illness, and other grand-scale social problems. What matters to him instead is to understand this illness from the perspective of the individuals struggling with it on a daily, even minute-by-minute, basis—how it feels, what it means, how a person copes with it, how it shapes their interactions with others, and so on. There is a considerable challenge in this emphasis, because, according to Karp, a symbolic interaction perspective on depression is almost completely absent from the research literature on the subject:

> *what struck me looking at the statistical data was, here were people writing about affective disorders, writing about a feeling disorder, and in nowhere in all of this stuff, was I hearing the feelings of the people who had the disorder. It struck me as just strange, a strange contradiction, that people were writing about feelings without hearing the feelings of the people they were trying to write about.*

It is the researcher's methodological perspective that leads him or her to select a given research design. Karp's methodological perspective leads him to inquire about the "lived experiences" of those suffering from depression. He selects in-depth interviews as his primary method because they allow him to pursue research questions that focus on understanding depression from the perspective of those afflicted. For instance, Karp observed, "most of my work in the context of the symbolic interaction point of view about things is that it's an effort to see and to bring to the page the complexity of a messy phenomenon." He feels that for this reason the in-depth qualitative interview "allows me to meet my goal, which is to bring to the reader a deeper understanding of an extremely complex matter, and I think to myself . . . what really would additional numbers bring to the books that are already written?" Although he considered gathering quantitative data, he mainly sees this type of data as "background" for his qualitative results.

## The Perils of Mixed Methods

Another issue that is important to reflect on before embarking on a mixed methods study revolves around a researcher's familiarity with both qualitative and quantitative research. Researchers must ask themselves whether they have the training and resources necessary to carry out a mixed methods study.

For qualitative researchers, including quantitative data may be time-consuming and difficult to do, especially if one lacks training in the gathering and analysis of such data. Are the benefits worth the investment? David Karp talks about his hesitancy to take on another research method in his own work.

> SHARLENE HESSE-BIBER: *When, if at all, might a qualitative researcher with a qualitative methodology think about using mixed methods?*

> DAVID KARP: *You know, in some ways it's a very uncomfortable question you're asking because . . . what it is you tell students and what you do yourself [may be different]. Because I walk into a methods class, and . . . it doesn't take more than about two hours into the semester to start talking about triangulation and multiple methods, and every method has strengths and every method has weaknesses. . . . But in the end, I'm always saying to the students that if you have the time and the energy and the money, and you want to get the best results in a piece of work, then you ought to have methods that complement each other . . . and that's the best way that research ought to proceed and, if you can do it, that's the way you ought to do it.*

> *And then I go off in my own life and I don't do much in the way of mixing methods and so, in some ways, the question makes me sort of uncomfortable. And . . . I think there are a couple of reasons I could mention [as to why I don't]. One is that I think . . . you develop [ways of working] with which you feel comfortable, and it's hard to break from that. . . . If you develop an expertise . . . with the way you're doing things where you feel comfortable, where you've pulled it off before . . . it's hard, it takes a certain courage to stray from . . . what you do well, what's gotten you applause, and to start in some sense fooling around with [new] types of data. . . . It takes a little bit of a leap of courage . . . and maybe . . . a second dimension of this [is that] you haven't challenged yourself to integrate that kind of data into the writing that you do. It's partly a writing issue, I mean you get used to a certain kind of writing.*

Jumping on the mixed methods bandwagon without really thinking through the implications of doing so may yield research of dubious quality or research that does not add theoretical value and understanding to a research project. A quantitative researcher who lacks a basic understanding of qualitative methods but decides to use a qualitative method in his or her project runs the risk of "adding and stirring" his or her qualitative findings into a quantitative project. For example, in order to satisfy a funding agency that prefers a mixed method approach, a quantitative researcher might add a qualitative component to a study by including a few open-ended questions at the end of a (quantitative) survey. Karp described this approach, when used poorly or without theoretical purpose, as "sprinkling." Karp expanded on this point:

> And you know, if you read work where a method is just a throw in, it's just like going to the ice cream store and throwing a few M&Ms onto the top of the ice cream to make it look pretty, and it might taste a little bit better. When I see work like that, where the qualitative stuff is just thrown in for purposes of meeting an agenda, that doesn't really forward your understanding of the phenomenon or forward your theoretical thinking, that bothers me. I think all you're doing is being pragmatic and sort of following someone else's rules and falling in.
>
> I think we should use these methods when they can really forward our understanding, I mean truly forward our understanding of things theoretically, and any other reason strikes me as being problematic and in fact weakening the research that people do.

## The Practice of Mixed Methods:
## Behind the Scenes with Stephen Borgatti

Stephen Borgatti is a professor of Management. He is both an anthropologist and a mathematician and is particularly interested in social network analysis. He conducts qualitative and quantitative research projects, as well as mixed methods projects. I talked with him on the importance of the link between one's research problem and one's method and some of the issues researchers may face when the fit between the two does not work. Borgatti is especially skeptical of forcing premade research designs into your research project. He believes that mixing qualitative and quantitative methods can be very productive, and he does this regularly in his own work:

> If I do a network analysis, I typically am going to do some kind of ethnography first to find out what even are the right questions or, if it's theoretically driven, I know what questions I want to ask, I still have to know what language to use so they will understand the questions that I'm asking. So I do a little ethnography, to try to understand what's what, construct a sur-

*vey, then have people fill it out, and then, in the analysis, go back to people and say, "I'm finding this. How does this make sense to you, how do you interpret this picture?"*

However, Borgatti believes that the growing movement among funding agencies to require the addition of a qualitative component to their quantitative studies—a form of mixed methods design—is misguided. He referred to this approach of force-fitting research design into a predetermined mold as a form of "scientism" and "magical thinking" in which "the form of [the research] makes it scientific." Borgatti noted that this problem can also work in reverse, such that quantitative methods are force-fit into a primarily qualitative design simply to increase the apparent legitimacy of the research:

*I once saw a presentation by a postmodernist; he had done a factor analysis. And he put up these numbers and it was really interesting because it was sort of like a work of art, and the numbers were interpreted almost like a Rorschach, it [showed] little understanding about what factor analysis would involve. It was more like, I don't know, it was more like totems of some kind that he pulled out. . . . I think . . . he was doing it to add legitimacy to what he was doing. . . . He already had certain beliefs, and so he used the numbers to try to illustrate them, but the numbers weren't telling the conclusions. He wasn't drawing conclusions from the numbers. It was the other way around.*

## The Promise of Mixed Methods Research

An awareness of the importance of not "placing the cart before the horse" in mixed methods practice by centering the research problem holds the promise of enhancing existing theories and the discovery of new theoretical avenues. It is important that the research we do and the resulting data we collect relate back to our theoretical perspectives. Mixing methods can be an exciting process that might open our eyes to new realities and levels of understanding, but such a research design must be utilized only with the certainty that it will aid in "advancing our theoretical understanding" and not detract from our existing methodologies.

My own mixed methods journey began many years ago when I first thought about writing a mixed methods book. In keeping with the importance of knowing your researcher standpoint as we go forward on this journey, the following are a few reflections on my book-writing journey.

*My best recollection is that it all began as a nagging pain in the back of my mind each time I read articles and overall discussions about mixed methods by those whose reputations have been made in promoting these ideas. I am not the creator of this new wave of mixed methods.*

*I am a feminist qualitative researcher who has a particular perspective on social reality. As a feminist, I am interested in asking a set of research questions that often trouble the waters of traditional knowledge building by including issues of difference in the research process.*

*I am interested in issues of power, authority, and control while conducting research as well as asking such questions as: What is studied? From whose perspective? Who is being studied? Who is left out and needs to be included in this study? I guess you might say that I am a methods interloper—an outsider and an insider to mixed methods research.*

*As a sociologist who has had traditional training in quantitative methods and the positivist paradigm, I am an insider in that I practice and teach both methods and have in fact conducted several mixed methods projects. As a feminist, I am often the outsider who asks new questions, yet I will utilize a range of tools—quantitative and qualitative—as needed to answer my questions. I am not wedded to one specific method or set of methods. I use whatever methods will facilitate getting answers to my research problem(s).*

*As a researcher, my agenda is one of promoting a comprehensive approach and understanding of the use of methods techniques by placing the practice of methods more firmly within a research context. If we are to realize the potential synergy of a mixed methods approach, it is important to understand the interconnections and philosophical groundings that connect our methods to research problems. I am cognizant of the importance of living within the contradictions and tensions of the research process. I enter into dialogue with this process. To dialogue means confronting our assumptions, suspending judgment, and embracing difference. To dialogue also means to hone our listening skills, with a stance toward understanding. I decided to write this book with the goal of providing researchers with a user-friendly guide to the practice of a qualitative approach to mixed methods research.*

SHARLENE HESSE-BIBER

## GLOSSARY

**complementarity:** one of the reasons for using mixed methods; accomplished by utilizing both quantitative and qualitative data to understand the social story, allowing the researcher to gain a fuller understanding of the research problem and/or clarify a given research result.

**critical/postmodernist theories:** qualitative approaches that examine how social life is produced and the privileges given to those in power, with a goal to emancipate and to expose social injustice.

**development:** aided by mixed methods when the "results from one method . . . help develop or inform the other method" (Greene et al., 1989, p. 259).

**expansion:** a reason for doing mixed methods research; used to "extend the breadth and range of the inquiry" (Greene et al., 1989, p. 259).

**feminist approach:** is specifically interested in understanding knowledge "for women"; moves the issues of those whose lives have been marginalized, overlooked, or misrepresented by traditional investigations to the front and center of the research agenda.

**initiation:** use of mixed methods leads to findings that raise questions or contradictions that will require clarification, thus initiating a new study.

**interpretative approach:** researcher's epistemology assumes multiple subjective realities that consist of stories or meanings produced or constructed by individuals within their "natural" settings.

**intersectionality:** refers to standpoints or worldviews created by the overlapping of a combination of locations within the social structure (i.e., race, class, gender, sexuality, geography, etc.).

**methods triangulation:** a reason for using mixed methods; the use of more than one method while studying the same research question. The researcher is looking for a convergence of the data collected by all employed methods in a study to enhance the credibility of the research findings.

**mixed methods:** a research design that uses both quantitative and qualitative data to answer a particular question or set of questions.

**positivism:** the central belief that there exists an objective reality and that "facts" are independent of any individual's subjective experience and values.

**standpoint theory:** the argument that a woman's oppressed locations within society provides fuller insights into society as a whole; standpoint theorists stress the necessity of starting research from women's lives.

**subjugated knowledge:** the knowledge of oppressed groups that has often been left out of or ignored in traditional research and mainstream research inquiry.

---

## DISCUSSION QUESTIONS

1. What factors have contributed to the growth of mixed methods research? Additionally, how does this relate to the exposition of subjugated knowledge?

2. What is the difference between mixed methods and multimethods?

3. For what reasons should you use a mixed methods approach?

4. How does the current mixed methods approach ignore methodology, and why is this problematic?

5. What are the benefits of using a qualitative mixed methods approach?

6. What are some of the problems with using a mixed methods approach?

---

## ■ ■ ■ SUGGESTED WEBSITES ■ ■ ■

### Mixed Methods Research

*www.socialresearchmethods.net/tutorial/Sydenstricker/bolsa.html*

Provides information about mixed methods within the context of a specific case study/tutorial.

*mmr.sagepub.com*

The *Journal of Mixed Methods Research*, started in 2007, is an excellent source of research on mixed methods that covers empirical mixed methods studies and discussions of epistemological and methodological issues in the field of mixed methods.

## NOTE

1. For a fuller account of the contemporary work on mixed methods research, see Bergman (2008); Bryman (1988); Creswell (1998, 2006, 2008); Creswell and Plano Clark (2008); Greene (2007); Greene and Caracelli (1997); Morgan (1998); Sandelowski (2000a); Sieber (1973); Tashakkori and Teddlie (1998, 2003); and Teddlie and Tashakkori (2008).

2. All excerpts from Kantor (2007). Copyright 2007 by The New York Times. Reprinted by permission. All rights reserved.

# CHAPTER 2

# Formulating Questions, Conducting a Literature Review, Sampling Design, and the Centrality of Ethics in Mixed Methods Research

This chapter addresses the art of asking questions in a mixed methods research design and the link between asking questions and the selection of research methods. What types of methods, analyses, and interpretations are brought to bear in understanding a given set of research questions? In line with our comprehensive approach to mixed methods, we look at the critical role that researcher reflexivity plays in guiding the researcher through the question-asking stage of the research process. We also discuss the influence of relevant stakeholders (granting agencies and researcher sponsors), the role of the literature review, and even the occurrence of serendipity in shaping the question-asking process. We examine mixed methods sampling strategies that are often left out of mixed methods discussions. Finally, we discuss the centrality of ethics in the research process.

## Researcher Reflexivity in the Question-Asking Process: The "Cart before the Horse" Metaphor

The metaphor of the "cart before the horse" is a cautionary one in that it reminds us of a tendency to let our methods focus sometimes turn into the driving force in our research projects. An understanding of our own research standpoints as we embark on mixed methods research projects may serve to offset this tendency. Of course, our methods decisions interact not only with our research questions but also with the skills and resources we bring to the research endeavor, as I comment on later in this chapter. Even so, we should also remain cognizant of the fact that our values, attitudes, and biases play an important role in determining (1) what questions we ask or do not ask, (2) what type of data we collect, and (3) the type of method, analysis, and interpretation that shapes our understanding of the research problem. The research question is pivotal in guiding the type of mixed methods analysis and interpretation that a researcher pursues, as well as the overall design of her or his research project. Figure 2.1 shows the linkages between these elements. Research questions imply a worldview or theoretical perspective that is either conscious (the solid arrow) or unconscious (the broken arrow).

A researcher's worldview affects his or her standpoint and approach to research. Lynne Giddings talks about the importance of knowing one's standpoint in the research process, especially for novice mixed methods researchers. This is important, as one might unconsciously follow the dominant paradigm of his or her discipline without a critical assessment of the values and attitudes of a particular discipline's paradigmatic view. Giddings (2006) wrote:

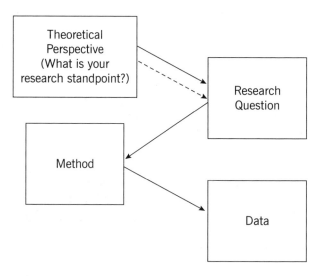

**FIGURE 2.1.** Relationship of theoretical framework to research, method, and data collection.

Although the novice may not yet know the language and processes of research, they already know in part the research culture they are entering. Unless students have experienced being different from the cultural mainstream, the equation of research with science is not questioned; the beliefs, values and attitudes that go along with it are taken for granted. . . . What the novice researcher is learning is the "ready made thinking" . . . of their discipline's research. They learn that methodologies from certain paradigms hold more value than others. (p. 200)

Also underlying a researcher's methodological preferences is a set of value assumptions, or *axiology*, that we bring to social inquiry from our own lives (Lincoln & Guba, 1985, p. 37). Jennifer Greene (2002), for example, noted that certain methodologies are both sociopolitical and moral and that the field of evaluation research is particularly value laden. She observed:

Evaluation practice decisions are socio-political and moral decisions—precisely because our methodologies include value commitments and political stances—and . . . evaluators rarely have complete control over all of these practice decisions, notably including decisions about mixing methods. . . . Evaluation stakeholders appear to value the potential of multiple methods to facilitate interdisciplinary work or work that is more comprehensive. . . . When our evaluation practice decisions are constrained by sponsor politics and dictates, the possibilities of conducting a mixed-method study as we envision it are similarly constrained. (pp. 260–261)

Julianne Cheek is a Professor at the Institute of Nursing and Health Sciences at the University of Oslo and in the School of Health Sciences at the University of South Australia. A leading qualitative researcher, she addresses the importance of mixed methods researchers' remaining cognizant of the tight link between theory and research methods within a mixed methods project. Let's go behind the scenes with Julianne Cheek.

SHARLENE HESSE-BIBER: *What do you think about researchers who say you can't mix quantitative and qualitative research methods because they arise from two different paradigms and that's not acceptable on philosophical grounds?*

JULIANNE CHEEK: *I probably take the middle ground on this one. I know exactly where they're coming from, and I think they make a very good point. Some researchers are doing what I call "theoretical shopping." It is like when you pick out a packet of corn flakes and a packet of Cocoa Puffs and something else and you throw it all in the bowl and you say you've got mixed methods but you haven't really. . . . They're still totally bound by their assumptions and everything else. You know the assumption of "if I mix them more in the bowl somehow I'll get something that hangs together." Well, you and I both know that's not the case. I . . . think that the methods are very different in terms of their philosophy, the ontological and epistemological assumptions that sit underneath them.*

*I think that if you are going to include [qualitative and quantitative methods] in one study, you have to declare [your underlying assumptions] . . . you know, it is not just a matter of mixing some techniques, it's actually a matter of mixing some assumptions about knowledge, assumptions about the type of data . . . assumptions about the world we live in . . . and how you write that up. . . .*

Practicing reflexivity helps researchers get in touch with their research assumptions by making them more conscious of what values, attitudes, and research concerns they bring to a given research endeavor. Consider the following reflexive questions as you embark on your own mixed methods research project:

- How does your position in society affect the way you observe and perceive others in your daily life?

- What particular values and biases do you bring to and/or impose on your research?

- What particular ideas on the nature of knowledge/reality do you bring to your research?

- How do these ideas connect to the specific research questions and methods you employ in a research project?[1]

Sociologist David Karp illustrates the important connection between our worldview, the kinds of research questions we ask, and the methods we utilize. He observes that he is drawn to using a qualitative approach because of his intrinsic interest in the complexity, variation, and multifacetedness of the social world. This is a view of social reality that is harder to capture using correlation techniques that are best suited for demonstrating general (and generalizable) social trends and statistical averages, rather than complexity, uniqueness, and variability in social phenomenon. Here, Karp expands on his view:

*I'm interested in the messiness of things. I'm interested in life circumstances that are difficult, that are complicated, that are multifaceted, that don't allow for simple correlation regularities, law-like kinds of statements. And I think there are lots of social scientists who are afraid of messiness. They avoid messiness because the methods they are using are not designed . . . to deal with that messiness. What they're looking for are clear patterns. Now I'm looking for patterns, too. We're all looking for patterns. But I'm equally interested in . . . all the variations from the patterns. Because there is no one single story. . . . I think that my little experience with the quantitative stuff that I read is that there is very little tolerance for that diversity and that ambiguity and so on.*

## The Influence of Stakeholders in the Formulation of Research Questions

Research is not conducted in a vacuum, and many researchers must consider the concerns and interests of individuals or groups that provide funding and resources or that have another claim on the project. The interests of these *stakeholders* can influence, to varying degrees, the direction a project takes (see Figure 2.2). As such, it is important to ask ourselves an additional reflexive question:

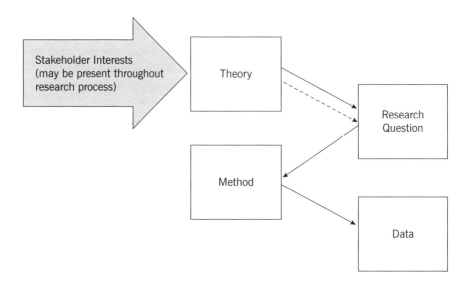

**FIGURE 2.2.** The influence of stakeholders in the formation of research questions.

- To what extent is my research project constrained or supported by other stakeholders (e.g., granting agencies and researcher sponsors)?

A range of stakeholder interests can shape a particular research question. A researcher may pursue a particular topic and setting because there is funding available to study that issue. Granting agencies are either public (i.e., national and international), private (i.e., foundations), or corporate (public and private), and these groups dispense funds to study specific societal issues and therefore can influence the direction a research project may take. Bryman (2007b) interviewed a purposive sample of 20 social scientists and specifically asked them about their mixed methods research practices. In addition, he perused the literature on published mixed methods research to ascertain how researchers talked about the connection between the problem and the mixed methods they utilized in their research. These interviews reveal that there are strategic factors other than the research problem that researchers take into account in selecting a particular research question, and one of these factors is stakeholder interests.

Bryman (2007b) noted that not only do stakeholder interests shape the research question, but these interests also affect the methods selected. In fact, he noted that sometimes the relationship between the problem and method is "spurious" in that stakeholder interests only make it seem as if the problem and method are in fact related:

> The way research questions are formulated and how data are collected and analysed are influenced by researchers' beliefs about the following: disciplinary requirements concerning what should pass as acceptable knowledge; policy makers' expectations concerning the kind of knowledge they require for policy; and expectations of funding bodies. (p. 16)

A good example of the issue of stakeholder influence comes from studying the history of Arctic science research, in which a review of research projects reveals a bias toward dominant societal interests. In this example, stakeholders from the "dominant society" hold real power in determining the focus and direction of research projects:

> The history of Arctic science has, for the most part, been written by individuals who were or are part of what might be called the "dominant society" and it generally reflects the views, insights, biases, and

epistemology of the dominant society . . . other views, particularly of any society with oral traditions, are not documented in written form. As an example, the research agendas proposed by the Northwest Territories and Nunavut (Canada) were once strongly social and cultural, while they have now moved towards distinctive economic orientations. Central governments have tended to emphasize sovereignty, the national interest, and the large resource economy. Priorities have fluctuated with the Cold War, energy security, and terrorism. (ICARP II, 2005, pp. 6–11)

Arctic research challenges us to look at who benefits from the asking of a particular question. It is clear that indigenous peoples are often left out of the question-making equation, whereas those stakeholders holding strong economic, national, and international interests influence the types of questions asked in this study area and, indeed, in many other areas as well. If there is a commitment to including community members in the research project, the asking of questions becomes more complex, as the number of stakeholders involved in the research project expands. Some exemplary research projects demonstrate how to consciously incorporate multiple stakeholder concerns, including the voices of those living in the research community under study (see Westhues et al., 2008).

What is important to consider is that there is a social, political, and economic dimension to the asking of research questions, and it is important that we interrogate all these levels, including our unique values and motives, in the question-making process.

## The Role of the Research Literature[2]

Reviewing research literature is often an important means of devising research questions (see Figure 2.3). Although initial interest may spur us on to a particular research area, the specific aspects of the problem we want to focus on may not be so clear. In many ways, the literature review can be the compass that guides your research. If you begin a project with a vague understanding of your topic, you can conduct a review of research literature to narrow down the possibilities to be included under the umbrella of your study. This is particularly helpful with the advent of computerized research tools. Becoming acquainted with basic retrieval systems for literature can be instrumental in the early steps of your research. Many databases available on- and offline can

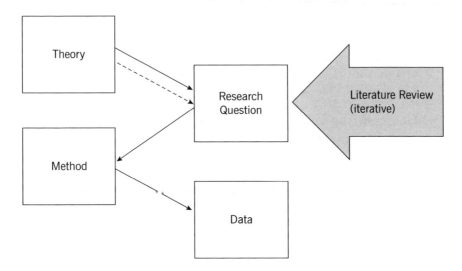

**FIGURE 2.3.** The role of research literature in the formulation of research questions.

help you formulate the basic foundation of your research, and many of these databases offer full article abstracts and reports online. This puts a wealth of research right at your fingertips, and focusing the scope of your literature review (and thus your research project) becomes that much easier with these tools.

Beginning with a few *key terms* might also be helpful for narrowing your literature review in the early steps of the project. Considering phrases and terms that are pivotal to your proposed topic would narrow your search field, and considering the motives and techniques of article authors is helpful. Peruse the information in these databases with a careful eye, and do not be afraid to ask yourself important questions that will enlighten your understanding of the articles.

### The Basics of a Literature Review

The literature review should frame the context of your specific research problem. In other words, it should provide a "rationale" for the selection of your particular research problem. The literature review does this by showing the reader that you have knowledge of your research problem and understand the critical theoretical and research issues that are contained in your research problem. The literature review should not be a summary of all the literature on your research topic, but it should be a critical evaluation of what you consider the relevant literature on your specific research problem. The reader should have a good idea of the range of viewpoints on your problem.

### Writing Up Your Literature Review

Your literature review should integrate findings and come up with a critical evaluation and/or synthesis of the literature on your mixed methods research problem. You will need to briefly describe for the reader how you went about gathering literature on your research problem. Did you consult databases? Did you seek a range of literature on your specific problem? Was the literature you found well reasoned and legitimate?

Another goal of the literature review is to show your reader that your research will make a significant contribution to the field. There are a variety of strategies that you can utilize to accomplish this goal.

- You might show the reader that there is a significant gap in the current understanding of your research problem.

- You might show the reader that your research problem will help to resolve or extend an important theoretical understanding and/or that you have created a new model for understanding the research problem under study.

As you gather the literature on the topic, you should keep in mind other details that have to do with the content and format of your literature review. Refer to the most current literature on your research problem, and be sure to include key readings, whether current or classic, on your research problem. Also, it is preferable to turn to primary sources as opposed to secondary data sources; always return to the primary source, as any issues that arise can more clearly be elucidated in a "conversation" with a primary text or project. It is important to make sure that all your sources are valid and reliable; this is especially true with data obtained from the Internet, as it can be difficult to distinguish credible articles and papers from less reputable sources. Online journal articles in particular can be misleading; make sure that the journal articles you use are peer reviewed.

Additionally, a literature review should be focused and not repetitive. Often, academic articles, referencing other sources, repeat the same ideas. Although all these works are important to the larger scholarship in a given area, you need not reiterate one idea, theory, or finding multiple times just to show its validity. Remember, a literature review grounds the foundation of your research, but it is not the sole focus of your research endeavor. It is a framework upon which your research rests, and although it needs to be reliable, accurate, and well written, it need not be the bulk of your finished article or publication.

In addition to helping one to formulate a research question, a literature review can guide and focus the early steps of your research. Knowing how to develop a literature review, as well as recognizing its potential benefits, is a critical part of embarking on a successful mixed methods research project. Locke, Spirduso, and Silverman (2007) created a helpful metaphor for us to consider when approaching the literature review process. These researchers suggested approaching the literature review like an "extended conversation":

> The process of locating the voices of individual conversants, for example, is called *retrieval*. That involves searching through the accumulated archive of literature to find out what has been said (when, by whom, and on the basis of what evidence). The process of listening carefully to the ongoing discourse about a topic of inquiry is called *review*. That involves studying items previously retrieved until both the history and the current state of the conversation are understood. (Locke et al., 2007, pp. 63–64)

### Mixed Methods Literature Reviews

Much of the literature review work for a quantitatively driven mixed methods study is conducted up front for the research project. This type of literature review is more extensive and focused so as to fully justify the testing of particular hypotheses that emanate directly from your research problem. The literature review does not have to be as extensive at the beginning of a qualitatively driven mixed methods project because, once out in the field, the research questions shift often due to the discovery-oriented nature of a qualitative approach to research. Given the iterative nature of a qualitative approach to mixed methods, a researcher will often find that he or she is referring back to the literature at different points throughout the analysis of the data in order to help place the research findings in a wider context. Furthermore, the literature he or she refers back to may shift as the focus of the research shifts. For example, a researcher may have originally done an extensive literature review on eating disorders among college-age women, but, after beginning a study in the field on women with eating disorders, the researcher may shift his or her focus to specifically looking at how black women deal with eating disorders. He or she must then research and confront a whole new area of literature on the topic of black women and eating disorders.

We can think of the qualitatively driven mixed methods approach literature review as a process whereby the research literature is woven throughout the research project. The literature should not be used to impose a point of view on the data but rather should function as a "consultant." For example, a researcher might examine the literature to see whether his or her particular research findings are supported by the literature (triangulation). If he or she discovers that the findings differ, the research literature may offer some clues as to where he or she might proceed next or may provide some information about making sense of the anomalous findings.

You might consider the following questions as a checklist when reviewing literature for a mixed methods project:

- How are topics defined in the research?

- What key terms and phrases do authors employ?

- How have other researchers approached the topic?

- What controversies emerge in the literature?

- What are the most important findings from this literature?

- What findings seem most relevant to your interests?

- What pressing questions still need to be addressed concerning your topic?

- Are there gaps in the literature?

We now return to the topic of formulating research questions in a mixed methods project.

# Types of Research Questions

## Methods-Centric Questions

Researchers often devise research questions that are difficult to research because of money and time constraints. While not sacrificing his interest in understanding the dynamics of classroom learning, James A. Banks (1976) negotiated his research interests in urban education when he pursued a research question with cost-effective and time-efficient methodology. He decided on the following question: How are black Americans depicted in textbooks?

> My first idea for a Ph.D. research project was to study the effects of an experimental training program on the attitudes and beliefs of teachers in urban schools. I had to abandon this idea for several reasons. First, it was necessary that I complete my study within a one-year period, and it was unlikely that I would have been able to design and implement the kind of study I had in mind within those limitations. Second, I needed the cooperation of a large urban school district and numerous teachers to conduct the study, and the initial response I received from one large city school district convinced me that it was unwilling to cooperate with me in implementing the study. Third, the study would have been quite expensive to conduct, and I did not have the funds to finance this type of research project. Although I was disappointed because I was unable to implement my "ideal" study, I did not despair. I realized that although the classroom teacher is the most important factor in the child's learning environment, there are other variables that influence student mastery of content and acquisition of attitudes. Of these other variables, the textbook was perhaps the most important. (Banks, 1976, pp. 383–384)

Banks was cognizant of the important link between the research question and the method. The context of constraints forced him to negotiate his problem and set upon an unobtrusive research project that consisted of conducting a content analysis study of how black Americans were portrayed in mainstream educational textbooks. The selection of a research method that cut down on his initial time and money constraints was primary, yet he still maintained a tight link between the problem and the method by shifting his problem focus to one that was amenable to a content analysis inquiry.

In some cases, however, the preference for a given method may serve to dictate the specific data collected and the problem we study. Figure 2.4 depicts this methods-driven approach.

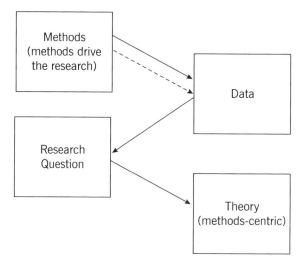

**FIGURE 2.4.** Methods-centric approach in the formulation of research questions.

In another example, Anthony Dobb and Alan Gross (1976) wanted to study the psychological phenomenon of frustration. However, they already knew that they wanted to use a particular method in their study, namely, an unobtrusive method that would allow them to study research participants without the participants' knowing they were being studied. Because they began with a chosen method, the method was what guided the development of their research question and subsequent data collection. They note this methods-driven approach as follows:

> Most social science research looks as if it were planned in a straightforward, logical fashion. Reports are written as if the people involved had just finished reading the relevant literature and saw a need for a particular question to be answered. It generally looks as if these scientists thought a great deal about the best way to answer the question and then designed their research accordingly. [Our] research . . . does not conform to this pattern. Instead, it resulted from an explicit, self-conscious attempt to design a study utilizing a specific method, which, at the time, was relatively underused in psychology. In fact, in this case, the content that was eventually studied [horn honking] was selected only because it was amenable to the method of interest. (Dobb & Gross, 1976, p. 487)

Studying horn honking (an unobtrusive measure) within a natural (unconstructed) setting allowed Dobb and Gross to form an experiment in which they measured an individual's level of frustration as linked to the number and frequency of horn honks:

> We thought about a number of different ways to frustrate people, eventually thinking about one of the day-to-day frustrations that most urban people experience, that of traffic jams . . . it did not take long until one of us . . . realized that it is easy to frustrate someone in traffic simply by not moving when a traffic light turns green. In a few minutes, then, we had developed our ideas for our dependent variable. . . . We would simply time how long it would take for the driver behind us in line to honk his or her horn. (Dobb & Gross, 1976, p. 488)

What we can observe from assessing some of the factors and influences that shape our research interests and the specific research questions we address is multidimensional. Having said this, once a question is settled on, it behooves the researcher to be mindful of the linkage between problem and method. What types of research questions lend themselves to a mixed methods approach? In tackling this question, let's start by understanding what a quantitative approach to question asking entails and what a qualitative approach to question formulation requires.

### Differences between Qualitative and Quantitative Research Questions

Quantitative and qualitative approaches to research have their own ways of structuring the research problem. It is important that we are aware that, once we buy into a particular research approach, the approach will have its own language of inquiry. Let's look at the structuring of a quantitative and qualitative approach in the formulation of a research question or set of questions. In the next sections, we look specifically at the type of research questions that tend to "fit" with a particular research methods approach.

Gubrium and Holstein (1997) noted that qualitative researchers raise "what" and "how" questions:

> The commanding focus of much qualitative research is on questions such as *what* is happening, *what* are people doing, and *what* does it mean to them? The questions address the content of meaning, as

articulated through social interaction and as mediated by culture. The resulting research mandate is to describe reality in terms of what it naturally is. (Gubrium & Holstein, 1997, p. 14)

"What" questions address the nature of individual action in social settings, "looking for the meanings that exist in, emerge from, and are consequential for, those settings" (p. 14). For example, asking questions such as, What are students' perceptions of the new grading system recently implemented at their college? How do students perceive their Facebook online friendships? Focus on the construction of meaning from the perspective of those within a social setting: "*how* questions typically emphasize the production of meaning. Research orients to the everyday practices through which the meaningful realities of everyday life are constituted and sustained. The guiding question is *how* are the realities of everyday life accomplished?" (Gubrium & Holstein, 1997, p. 14).

Through the asking of "what" and "how" questions, qualitative researchers explore the specific dynamics or processes of everyday life. These questions focus on a specific social context, and these processes and dynamics are often difficult to quantify and often remain hidden.

Quantitative questions are stated in the form of testable hypotheses—predicting the possible outcome of a relationship between two or more variables, one that is independent (assumed to be the cause) and the other dependent (assumed to be the effect or outcome). For example, the deductive question regarding the increases in obesity rates among adolescents we addressed earlier might be framed as follows:

- Hypothesis 1: There is a relationship between gender (independent variable) and obesity (dependent variable) rates among children.

- Hypothesis 2: Adolescent girls will have higher obesity rates compared with adolescent boys.

Often quantitative questions can take on some of the following formats (not exhaustive):

- To what extent does $X$ cause a change in $Y$?

- To what extent is $X$ associated with $Y$?

- If $X$, then $Y$?

# What Are Mixed Methods Research Questions?

The field of mixed methods research contains a paucity of literature on how to ask mixed methods questions. In a recent review of the mixed methods literature, Onwuegbuzie and Leech (2006) noted the lack of attention given to formulating mixed methods questions and the pivotal role that they play in the mixed methods research process. They stated:

> It is surprising that an extensive review of the literature revealed no guidance as to how to write research questions specifically in mixed methods studies. The leading textbook in mixed methods research, *Handbook of Mixed Methods in Social and Behavioral Research* (Tashakkori & Teddlie, 2003) . . . does not provide any significant discussion of research questions in mixed methods research. In fact, nowhere in this 768-page, 26-chapter edited book is the concept of mixed methods research questions either defined or described. (Onwuegbuzie & Leech, 2006, p. 477)

The simple answer to the question, "What are mixed methods research questions?" is that they are questions that require the use of both quantitative and qualitative methods to answer the question or set of questions.[3] Yet to make sure that a mixed methods research design enhances our theoretical understanding, it is useful to look at some of the factors involved in the mixed methods question-asking process.

### The Question-Asking Process in Mixed Methods Research

It is important to ask yourself if your research question stems from the same theoretical/methodological framework or from different frameworks. What theoretical frameworks do you bring to this particular mixed methods question, and are you conscious of your own theoretical frameworks and biases? The question-making process in mixed methods research works well when the researcher is cognizant of his or her research standpoint and allows this standpoint to guide the process. Researchers may have a good idea beforehand of what questions they want to ask when they decide to mix methods at the data collection stage. Sometimes the methods are employed sequentially (one, then the other) and sometimes concurrently (at the same time). There is a deliberate quality to the research design and a sense of what each method can contribute to answering the overall set of research questions. In addition to this, a variety of factors may intervene between your stated research question and the question or set of mixed methods questions you wind up addressing in your final project.

### The "Serendipity" Factor in the Question-Asking Process

Sometimes a mixed methods question arises in a serendipitous manner simply because the initial data collection and analysis using one particular method raise more questions than the original method can answer. In these cases, the research questions may need to be reviewed and/or an additional research method may be required to answer the question. Such is the following scenario: A researcher has a research problem that does not necessarily appear to lend itself to a mixed methods design. In this case, the question is, "What is the relationship between adolescent obesity and poverty?"

The goal is to understand whether there is a causal relationship between poverty and rates of obesity in adolescents. Such a question would seem to require the use of large-scale survey data to test whether or not there is a causal relationship between poverty (independent variable) and obesity (dependent variable). Researchers Wang and Beydouns (2007) suggested that such a relationship exists. Yet researchers may find that they need to ask a series of additional questions, as the initial findings from their quantitative study calls forth a set of "why" questions, first and foremost of these being, Why are the poor often obese? The asking of this question leads to another process factor, that of *iteration*.

### The "Iterative" Factor in the Mixed Methods Research Question-Asking Process

New "why" questions sparked by findings from the original study may require the researcher to shift his or her methodological standpoint if the goal is to explore and understand the lived experiences of those individuals who are poor and obese. Although the original findings showed that poverty is related to obesity, the relationship was found to be more complex, as other factors such as minority status, ethnicity, and gender also appeared to play a complex part in understanding adolescent obesity in the findings. Yet these factors of influence are at a variable level of understanding; we still do not know why low-income children, especially those from certain racial, ethnic, and/or gender groups, have higher rates of obesity. What is it about the experience of those who reside in low-income areas that places them at a higher risk for obesity? These "why" questions lead researchers to collect data using a qualitative method, which requires the use of intensive interviews or semistructured interviews to ask in-depth questions about the social context of obesity.

From this one example, we can see that the asking of questions itself takes on an iterative form such that the asking of one question leads to the asking of several other questions. The question-making process interacts with empirical data in a spiral that moves back and forth between the research question, methods, data analysis and findings, and so on, moving toward a more complex set of new questions (see Figure 2.5).

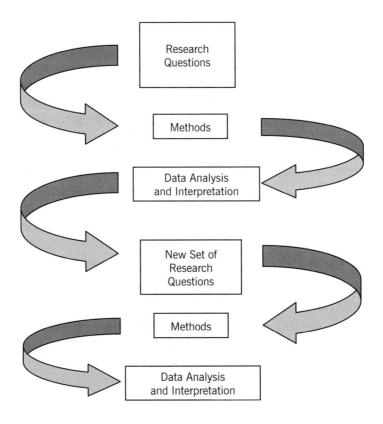

**FIGURE 2.5.** Interaction between methods and data in formulating research questions.

### The "Researcher's Standpoint" as a Factor in the Question-Asking Process

As the question begins to shift from "Is there a relationship between *X* and *Y*?" to "What is the lived experience of *X* and *Y*?" we have mixed methods and started to mix methodologies. Each of these questions stems from a different type of theoretical understanding of social reality. The first question seeks generalizations and uses methods to get at social facts. Essentially, the idea is that there is a number out there that will reveal whether the rates of obesity are higher for some groups than others.

Understanding at this level of variable analysis is based on statistical difference and causal modeling. A researcher with a positivistic approach might study rates of obesity, for example, between poor and nonpoor individuals and explore which specific factors associated with poverty lead to obesity. However, another researcher might want to explore the experiential or phenomenological aspects of obesity among the poor by asking, "How can we understand what it is like to live with the stigma of being poor and obese?" This is a different question, one that begins to shift our theoretical focus from the macro to the micro level, at which the goal is not to make generalized statements but to explore the social context within which these variable relationships arise. In making this shift in question asking, we are shifting our methodological or theoretical focus. In this case, there is a *methodological shift* in the researcher's standpoint that brings to light new questions that can also influence the type of methods we select.

## Returning to the "Cart before the Horse" Metaphor: A Caveat

Although the metaphor of "placing the cart before the horse" reminds us of the importance of the research problem in the methods design we select, it is also important not to be taken in by those who may use this metaphor to silence new ways of thinking about social reality. I am reminded here of a conference speech given by Nelson Mandela, then president of the African National Congress, to end apartheid in South Africa. He notes:

> Nearly 18 months ago when we met in Durban, we were striving to stave off all kinds of protestations among those who fear the people

and therefore fear democracy. We were being warned that elections
before a constitution is drafted would be to *put the cart before the horse*
[emphasis mine]. Others doubted whether the demand for a Constituent Assembly was in fact achievable.

We said yes, because we knew then as we know now that South
Africans have the capacity to bring about democracy.

Today, after a long and tortuous road, the National Party regime
has been forced to accept this reality. (Mandela, 1993)

Nelson Mandela's invocation of the "cart before the horse" metaphor is an important lesson for the practice of social research in that
it reminds us that sometimes entrenched metaphors seem like sound
reasoning, but they can also be used by those in power as justification
for stifling social change and disempowering those who seek social
change by asking new questions and seeking new solutions. It sometimes is prudent to turn this metaphor around and ask whether there
is, in fact, some wisdom in placing the cart before the horse in thinking about how research unfolds. Who should decide what the proper
linkage should be between any given cart and horse? Is it possible that
carts can tread where horses do not want to go? Must we always begin
with the horse? Mandela's visionary thinking and his courage are two
critical attributes among those whose research approaches call forth
new ways of thinking about social issues and whose goals are to create a more just society through social transformation. Placing the cart
before the horse must also be assessed within its given sociopolitical
context.

It is also important to remind ourselves that the research we do
does not occur in a vacuum. Textbooks such as this one present what
research might be in its form; however, we know that the practice is
different. Dilemmas arise in the conduct of research that prevent
the researcher from following his or her "ideal" problem → method
nexus. The example of methods-centric research cited earlier in this
chapter shows that in some contexts a methods-driven approach may
be most prudent or pragmatic. Social research, especially mixed methods research, exists in a turbulent environment, and the charge of the
researcher is to balance the ideals of research strategies with the day-
to-day contingencies and compromises that often accompany social
research practice. In addition, researchers must keep in mind that all
research is "from somewhere" and that all research has a point of view,
whether it is conscious or unconscious.

### Criteria for Evaluating a Mixed Methods Question

The following are some criteria for assessing the quality of your mixed methods research question.

- Is your question feasible? Can you, in fact, research this question? Do you have the time, money, and research skills to proceed to answer this question?

- Is the question ethical—that is, does it meet the standards of an institutional review board (IRB) ethics evaluation?

- Is the problem stated in a way that addresses the variety of different concerns/issues surrounding a given research problem?

- Is the research problem clearly stated and focused? For the quantitative component of the question, ask: Were the independent and dependent factors presented? Were hypotheses presented? Did the researcher define his or her main concepts?

- Is your question significant? There are a number of ways in which a research problem might be considered significant: Does the research problem add value to the existing literature? Does it suggest a new area for inquiry that looks promising? Does the research problem address an important research area in need of new knowledge?

Next, we discuss sampling designs, first looking at qualitative and quantitative designs and then at mixed methods approaches to sampling.

## Approaches to Sampling Designs

Qualitative and quantitative approaches to sampling design involve different assumptions about the nature of the social world. The goal of quantitative approaches is to ascertain specific "truths" about the social world with the goal of making generalizations. Quantitative approaches to sampling, therefore, need to ensure that their findings are representative of the general population under study. Quantitative sampling designs rely on "laws of probability" (the idea is that all members of a given population have an equal and known probability of being selected in a sample) in order to permit the use of statistical testing, so as to ascertain whether their research findings are in fact "true" with respect to their overall target population. There is a range of different types of probabilistic sampling designs.

■ *Simple random sample* (with or without replacement): Each member of the target population has an equal chance of being included in any given sample.

■ *Systematic random sample*: The researcher selects a sample from a randomly generated list that represents the target population (sampling frame). The researcher selects every *n*th element (the interval is determined by the size of the sample needed) from the list until the desired sample size is reached.

■ *Stratified random sample*: The researcher divides the target population into the desired groups (e.g., the population may be divided by social class) he or she wishes to sample from and then randomly selects population elements within each group until the target sample size is reached.

■ *Cluster sample and multistage cluster sample*: The target population is already divided into groupings, such as regions of the country, census tracts, neighborhoods, blocks, households, and so forth. The researcher may decide to sample within a given cluster (cluster sample) or across a range of clusters (multistage cluster sample). A multistage cluster sample of the U.S. population might involve first randomly selecting a sample of census tracts within different regions of the country; then, within each of the selected census tracts, randomly selecting blocks or clearly defined boundaries for rural areas; then within each of the blocks/areas, randomly selecting households; and, finally, within each household, randomly selecting a family member.

■ *Nonprobability convenience sampling*: Quantitative approaches also use nonprobability purposive samples; in this type of sample, the research question determines the type of elements selected in the sample. This sampling strategy is similar to nonprobability qualitative purposive sampling approaches.

### Qualitative Approaches to Sampling

Qualitative approaches have the goal of looking at a process, or subjective understanding. Qualitative samples are usually nonrandom and purposive or judgmental. The type of purposive sample will depend on the specific research question. Sometimes researchers will need a purposive sampling mix that consists of the most typical cases regarding a research problem; sometimes they will need the most extreme or deviant (outlier) cases. At other times, a research problem will call for selecting cases that represent either maximum diversity or sameness regarding a given problem. In a qualitative sampling procedure that follows a grounded theory approach, a "theoretical sampling" procedure is followed whereby the researcher decides who or what to sample next, based on prior data gathered from the same research project in order to make comparisons with previous findings (Glaser & Strauss, 1967). Analyses of findings in your current analysis of the data and the theoretical insights you come up with provide new sampling questions: Whom will I talk with next? What additional sources of data should I explore? What data will challenge or confirm my theoretical understanding of this finding (see Glaser & Strauss, 1967)? Sometimes, however, qualitative sampling does not follow a logical plan. Circumstance often provides the researcher with an *opportunistic sampling* possibility (Patton, 2002).

### Qualitative Approaches to Mixed Methods Sampling

Mixed methods sampling practice is conscious of the underlying research problems and recognizes that they are embedded in a given set of assumptions about the nature of the social world. Few mixed methods researchers discuss the issues involved in mixed methods sampling design. Collins, Onwuegbuzie, and Jiao's (2006) study of the prevalence of mixed methods sampling designs in social science research (they analyzed mixed methods studies that appeared in four leading school psychology journals between 2001 and 2004) and reported that the most common type of mixed methods sampling design consisted of a sequential design using multilevel samples (e.g., using students for the larger quantitative sample and teachers and/or administrators for the second, smaller qualitative sample). In addition, these researchers reported that in only a very small minority of these sequential studies was the qualitative component primary. For the most part, these research studies placed a greater emphasis on the results from the quantitative component, with the qualitative sample serving the quantitative (Collins et al., 2006, p. 97). What appeared most problematic in their perusal of these mixed methods studies is that 40% of them did not report their sample size, making it difficult to assess the statistical inferences that were made by the authors of these articles (Collins et al., 2006, p. 97). Collins and colleagues (2006) note:

The sample size omission is somewhat disturbing because it does not allow for the assessment of statistical power for any null hypothesis significance tests conducted in the quantitative phase . . . nor does it allow for a proper assessment as to the extent to which the quantitative findings are generalisable. . . . With respect to the qualitative phase, lack of information about the sample size makes it more difficult for the reader to determine the extent to which the researchers obtained data saturation. (pp. 97–98)

What seems even more problematic is that, in spite of the lack of sample size information, some of these mixed methods researchers proceeded to make unwarranted statistical generalizations (Collins et al., 2006, p. 98). What seems clear from this research study is that there are few guidelines about how mixed methods studies should be integrated, especially with regard to the types of generalizations one can make from these sampling designs (p. 98). What is also clear with regard to the results of this study is that the ideal sample size should flow from the specific research problem.

Onwuegbuzie and Collins (2007) have come up with a set of minimum sample size guidelines for qualitative and quantitative projects (see Table 2.1). For quantitative approaches to research, sample size is listed by the type of analysis that the researcher expects to carry out in her or his research project. We can note that for the three different analytical procedures (correlation, causal comparative analysis, and experimental analysis), different size samples are needed in order to run statistical tests to ascertain significance of findings. Table 2.1 also presents some of the most common qualitative research designs with minimum sample size recommendations adapted from Onwuegbuzie and Collins's (2007) research.

The particular mixed method sampling design chosen in a qualitative approach to mixed methods also depends on the research question. A qualitative research approach may employ a concurrent sampling design (QUAN + QUAL). In a concurrent sampling design, the samples from each study do not inform one another at the sampling stage; each sample is drawn separately. A concurrent sampling design may be employed by a qualitative researcher in order to increase the validity of her or his qualitative research findings with the goal of achieving agreement between the qualitative and quantitative findings.

A qualitative researcher may use a sequential sampling design in which the results of one study directly link with the next study. This can happen in a variety of sequential sampling designs. If the qualitative study has generated a specific set of theories, the researcher may then

**TABLE 2.1.** Minimum Sample Size Recommendations for Most Common Quantitative and Qualitative Research Designs

| Research design | Minimum sample size suggestions |
| --- | --- |
| Quantitative research design[a] | |
| Correlation analysis | 64 participants for one-tailed hypotheses; 82 participants for two-tailed hypotheses |
| Causal-comparative analysis | 51 participants per group for one-tailed hypotheses; 64 participants for two-tailed hypotheses |
| Experimental analysis | 21 participants per group for one-tailed hypotheses |
| Qualitative research design | |
| Case study | 3–5 participants |
| Phenomenological | 10 interviews |
| Grounded theory | 20–30 interviews |
| Ethnography | 1 cultural group; 30–50 interviews |

*Note.* Adapted from Onwuegbuzie and Collins (2007). Copyright 2007 by Nova Southeastern University. Adapted by permission.
[a]For correlational, causal-comparative, and experimental research designs, the recommended sample sizes represent those needed to detect a medium (using Cohen's [1988] criteria), one-tailed, statistically significant relationship or difference with .80 power at the .05 level of significance (Onwuegbuzie & Collins, 2007, p. 289).

seek to test out these generated ideas on a more representative population (QUAL → quan). A researcher may decide to use a sequential design employing a quantitative study first in order to gain perspective on what results seem important and worthy of further in-depth exploration (quan → QUAL). In addition, a qualitative researcher might employ a sequential design in order to increase the validity of his or her qualitative findings by using the quantitative sample to inform the specific type of qualitative sample chosen. For example, the findings from a quantitative sample can provide the criteria for deciding the particular population selected for a qualitative sample. In fact, the quantitative sample may provide the population from which a qualitative subsample is drawn, providing a direct link between the samples. The extent to which samples are directly linked, however, may raise some ethical concerns if in fact the identities of respondents from the quantitative sample are compromised in selecting the qualitative subsample for further in-depth research because informed consent has not previously been obtained from the respondents for a second study.

An excellent example of this type of direct-link sequential sampling design comes from a study by Nickel, Berger, Schmidt, and Plies (1995). In order to study sexual behavior and AIDS prevention among German adolescents, they carried out a sequential mixed methods sampling design. They interviewed a representative sample of 1,500 German adolescents ages 15–20. They conducted a statistical analysis of their findings, and, in addition, they performed a cluster analysis of these data, creating specific subpopulations with regard to their level of sexual experience. From these cluster groupings they randomly selected a subsample of individuals who represented the "most typical" respondent from each of the cluster groups and who were then interviewed in depth for the qualitative component of the project.

### Tips for Constructing Mixed Methods Sampling Designs

The following are some tips for ensuring that your mixed methods sampling design will adequately represent your intended research population and, in addition, will enhance the overall trustworthiness of your mixed methods research project.

1. The sampling design should flow from the research question. Is the goal of the study to test a hypothesis? To understand subjective experience? In pursuing these goals, other motivations may also arise in the study. In order to ensure that the study findings are valid, the researcher might employ a concurrent mixed methods design that contains both a qualitative and a quantitative sampling component. Or another motive might be to extend the research findings by employing a sequential mixed methods sampling design. Goals of and motivations for conducting a study play a prominent role in its overall sampling design.

2. Is the sample size adequate to answer the research problem and with regard to the overall research plan? If the researcher is interested in making generalizations to a wider target population from which a given sample is drawn, then a random sample with a specific size is required in order to statistically test for the significance of the research findings. If the research goal is to generate analytical significance, then an adequate number of cases is needed in order to achieve represen-

tation (saturation) of a given social phenomenon (see Morse, Onwuegbuzie & Collins, 2007).

3. To what extent does the sampling design allow the researcher to make specific conclusions regarding his or her mixed methods study? For example, if a researcher is making statistical generalizations, are they in fact warranted by the sampling design? If statistical generalizations are made from both the qualitative and quantitative findings to the target population, it is important that both the qualitative and the quantitative samples are chosen at random and from the same target population (see Collins, Onwuegbuzie, & Jiao, 2007; Onwuegbuzie & Johnson, 2006).

4. Do the sampling designs follow ethical guidelines set forth by such entities as the IRBs? This is especially important in sequential mixed methods designs in which the qualitative sample is drawn directly from the quantitative sample. Have all the participants in the quantitative study given their consent to also participate in a follow-up qualitative study?

This chapter concludes with a discussion of the ethical issues involved in conducting mixed methods research. Ethics is a critical element that runs through the research process, yet it is often a missing component in discussions of mixed methods practices.

## The Centrality of Ethics in the Mixed Methods Research Process[4]

Discussions of mixed methods research designs, like discussions concerning other research projects, often ignore or do not fully address the problem of ethics in social science research. Yet, in order to ensure the validity and accuracy of one's research, it is important for researchers to discuss ethical implications of their research and to remain conscious of moral integrity in their work. Hesse-Biber and Leavy (2006c) suggest the following questions researchers might consider before embarking upon their research projects:

- What moral principles guide your research?

- How do ethical issues enter into your selection of a research problem?

■ How do ethical issues affect how you conduct your research—the design of your study, your sampling procedure, and so forth?

■ What responsibility do you have toward your research participants? For example, do you have their informed consent to participate in your project? What ethical issues/dilemmas might come into play in deciding what research findings you publish? Will your research directly benefit those who participated in the study? (p. 86)

Ethical dilemmas do not cease to exist once your initial project proposal is approved by an ethics committee or IRB, whose job it is to oversee the ethical integrity of a research project. Ethics plays a role throughout the entire research process, and all researchers must be vigilant in checking themselves at every stage of their investigations. Self-monitoring your ethical standpoint is especially important with regard to mixed methods research projects, as these projects are more likely to contain thorny ethical issues that arise only after a project is under way. Beyond these general guidelines that are applicable for most research projects, mixed methods research designs harbor some specific ethical dilemmas that are particularly pronounced when researchers begin to integrate these methods at various stages of their ongoing projects. Let's look at a few potential ethical dilemmas that may arise at different stages of a mixed methods research project.

For example, a mixed methods sequential design that calls for using the personal (quantitative) data collected from a survey in order to obtain a sample for an in-depth qualitative study may result in inadvertently compromising a respondent's original informed consent and prior confidentiality agreements in this regard. For example, a researcher may violate a prior informed consent agreement by taking information from one study and using it as input for a (qualitative) component of another study without getting direct permission from the respondent to have his or her name used and identified as part of a sampling pool for that second, qualitative component. The use of respondents' information without their consent then becomes a direct invasion and violation of their privacy. In this case, it would be important for the researcher to ask respondents' permission to access their personal questionnaire data from the first study in order to conduct a follow-up study, if requested. Getting their consent to access these data may be impossible if the researcher is relying on secondary data that have already been collected.

Additional ethical issues arise from indirectly linking data in the
public domain in order to locate a target sample for further study. With
the advent of Internet technologies, for example, personal data are
already available online. Social networking sites such as Facebook and
MySpace, as well as global positioning systems (GPS) contain millions of
users whose personal information is in the public domain. Many of these
users of social networking software do not always appreciate that they are
revealing this information or understand the risks associated with making this type of private information readily available on the Web (Acquisti
& Gross, 2006; Bruce, 2007; Moreno, Fost, & Christakis, 2008).

Given the inherent nature of mixed methods linking of data, these
types of data can be particularly useful in targeting a purposive sample
and integrating information from studies of these sites to a qualitative
study. However, researchers must consider the following question: What
is the individual's right to privacy when personal data they put on a website for their friends and family can be linked to target them for all kinds
of reasons, including a mixed methods research project? Although some
social software has the capability to screen out interlopers, it is not fool-
proof, and some current research projects have already employed this type
of sampling technique in a range of different research projects (Boyd &
Ellison, 2007). Some current research projects, such as Boyd and Ellison's work on social networking sites, have addressed the range of privacy
concerns that have come about with the advent of Internet technologies.
Additionally, Hodge (2006) found that there is no legal precedent to deal
with the massive privacy issues that such sites pose. Who decides what
information on social network sites is off limits to third parties, and who
decides whether such information is in the public or private domain?

### Rethinking the Parameters of Informed Consent in Mixed Methods Research

These particular ethical issues are compounded and made more complicated in mixed methods research, and therefore we must pay careful attention to them. Early on, Brewer and Hunter (1989) advocated
caution in utilizing mixed methods, yet little about these ethical issues
is present in most current mixed methods discussions. Brewer and
Hunter stated:

> Researchers . . . need to make sure that their respondents are aware
> that the data they provide, say on a survey, may in fact be used in yet
> a second study and that in some cases, they may be re-contacted for

a follow-up interview. Yet . . . only a small portion of mixed methods researchers are in a position to obtain the informed consent to in fact carry out this type of research and the number of researchers conducting primary research projects is dwindling. . . . Two important and sweeping changes in the research environment have reduced the size of the subset of researchers eligible to use such mixed method designs. These include (1) an increase in the availability of secondary data and a corresponding decline in primary data collection efforts, and (2) increased awareness about data confidentiality and the protection of human research subjects. (1989, p. 151)

Researchers, then, need to be constantly on the lookout for ethically "sticky" situations and to explain their research practices explicitly in order to avoid controversies involving informed consent and improper use of confidential and "public domain" personal data. Establishing your ethical standpoint from the outset can help stem the ethical-issues tide that can easily rise in carrying out a mixed methods design. You might consider the following ethical guideline questions developed by Hesse-Biber and Leavy (2006c) as you proceed with your own mixed methods project:

- What types of ethical principles guide your work and life beyond the professional code of ethics you are bound by through a given discipline or professional association?

- Where do your ethical obligations to the researched start and end? (Hesse-Biber & Leavy, 2006c, p. 107)

- What ethical framework and philosophy informs your work and ensures respect and sensitivity for those you study, beyond whatever may be required by law? (adapted from Patton, 2002).

In addition to this set of questions, here are some other ethical questions to keep in mind as you proceed on your mixed methods research project:

- How will you communicate what your study is about to your research participants? How will you protect their privacy and emotional well-being during the course of the study? To what extent are you willing to press or extend the study?

- To what extent will you inform the research participant about your research aims? What steps will you take to establish informed consent?

■ Are you fully and properly meeting the requirements of your IRB and university guidelines, and are you comfortable with this level of confidentiality or interaction with your participants?

■ Will anyone other than you handle the data after the research is conducted? What can you do to assure your research participants of confidentiality or to fully inform them of potential uses for the material garnered?

The next chapter examines how research questions developed from a qualitative approach connect to mixed methods at the data analysis and interpretation stage of the research process. We look at the types of mixed methods designs that lend themselves to a qualitative research approach. We provide a set of guidelines about how one might link research questions with analytical and interpretative techniques. We also examine the role that computer-assisted qualitative data analysis software (CAQDAS) can play in assisting this linkage and provide some specific examples of how this might be done. We discuss some of the common issues raised in using such software tools to interpret and analyze mixed methods data.

## GLOSSARY

**axiology:** the study of the nature of value or value judgments.

**deductive questions:** questions cast in the form of testable hypotheses that state a relationship between two or more variables, one independent (assumed to be the cause) and the other dependent (assumed to be the effect or outcome).

**granting agencies**: public (i.e., national and international), private (i.e., foundations), or corporate (public and private) agencies that dispense funds to study specific research issues; they can influence the direction a research project may take.

**institutional review board:** a committee situated at a university or other research facility that oversees human research participants and seeks to protect their rights.

**iteration:** a repeating process; for example, the question-making process interacts with empirical data throughout the research project, moving toward a more complex set of new questions.

**key terms:** the phrases and terms pivotal to a proposed topic that can narrow down the search in a literature review.

**literature review:** the reading of all books, articles, and so forth relevant to the research topic; can help formulate a research question and focus the early steps of one's research.

**methodological shift:** a change in our methodological or theoretical focus; it can bring to light new questions that can also influence the type of methods we select.

**methods-driven approach:** the method chosen guides the development of the research question and subsequent data collection.

**reflexivity:** thinking about our research assumptions and becoming conscious of what values, attitudes, and concerns we bring to a given research project.

**retrieval:** the process within the literature review of locating the voices of individual conversers, which involves searching through the accumulated archive of literature to find out what has been said on one's research topic.

**stakeholders:** the people or organizations that have an interest in the results of a research project.

## DISCUSSION QUESTIONS

1. Explain the "cart before the horse" metaphor.

2. What kinds of reflexive questions should researchers ask themselves before beginning a project? How would you begin to answer these questions?

3. How do stakeholders influence research questions?

4. What are the benefits of a literature review for one's research project?

5. Discuss the differences between qualitative and quantitative research questions.

6. This chapter states that "the research we do doesn't occur in a vacuum." What does this mean?

7. Describe the ethical dilemmas that arise with the advent of social networking technology.

■ ■ ■ SUGGESTED WEBSITES ■ ■ ■

### Literature Reviews

*www.myunion.edu/library/litreview.asp*
*www.languages.ait.ac.th/EL21LIT.HTM*

These websites provide detailed information about literature reviews, including examples and additional suggested reading.

### Research Questions

*www.theresearchassistant.com/tutorial/2-1.asp*

This website is a guide to formulating a research question.

*www.esc.edu/esconline/across_esc/writerscomplex.nsf/0/f87fd7182f0ff21c-852569c2005a47b7*

This interactive website contains exercises in synthesizing research questions, such as honing in on the specificity of a certain topic of interest.

### The Qualitative–Quantitative Debate

*writing.colostate.edu/guides/research/observe/com2d3.cfm*

This website discusses the use of both quantitative and qualitative methods in mixed methods research, as well as their singular differences.

### NOTES

1. You might want to explore the following subquestions that derive from these four major reflexive queries: How do your intersecting social identities shape your worldview? What are your specific values and biases; for example, do you value the scientific method? Do you value social justice? Who do you believe can truly know about the topic in question? Does the researcher possess more information on the topic, or does the affected population have a clearer understanding of the phenomena that affect their lives? Do you take a more positivist approach to knowledge building and seek a unitary, objective reality that you believe is independent of subjective perception? To what extent, if any, do you assume the social world to consist of multiple, subjective, and socially constructed realities?

2. Parts of the sections "The Role of the Research Literature," and "Types of Research Questions" are adapted in part from Hesse-Biber and Leavy (2006f). Copyright 2006 by Sage Publications, Inc. Adapted by permission.

3. Here, we are employing the term "mixed methods" in its most common usage as a method that crosses the qualitative–quantitative divide. It must be noted, however, that researchers can mix two quantitative methods (surveys and experiments) or two qualitative methods (e.g., focus groups and intensive interviews).

4. This section is adapted in part from Hesse-Biber and Leavy (2006c). Copyright 2006 by Sage Publications, Inc. Adapted by permission.

# CHAPTER 3

# A Qualitative Approach to Mixed Methods Design, Analysis, Interpretation, Write Up, and Validity

## What Is a Qualitative Approach to Mixed Methods?

A qualitative approach to research encompasses several theoretical traditions. All of these approaches have the common core assumption that reality is socially constructed and that subjective meaning is a critical component of knowledge building. The qualitative tradition recognizes the importance of the subjective human creation of meaning but does not reject outright some notion of objectivity. Additionally, some qualitative perspectives stress a critical stance toward knowledge building, whereas others highlight the importance of transformation with an emphasis on social justice and social change as primary research objectives.[1]

The research method that qualitative researchers utilize often entails having a strong connection to one's research respondents through the practice of empathy, that is, by closely identifying with respondents' experiences. Individuals are perceived to be "meaning makers" of the worlds they reside in; it is their lived reality that qualitative researchers seek to understand. A qualitative approach does not place subjective experience outside the realm of scientific inquiry. Rather than seeking an answer to a given question with the goal of generalizing their findings to a wider population, qualitative researchers look for complexity. They value human subjectivity and seek to understand the range of experiences and the contexts within which they arise. Qualitative researchers often use both qualitative and quantitative methods in the service of a qualitative approach.

## A Mixed Methods Qualitative Framework

In general, a qualitative approach privileges qualitative methods, with the quantitative methods component playing an auxiliary role in a mixed methods framework (Howe, 2004, p. 54; see also Howe, 2003). Howe notes that such an approach also "actively engages stakeholder participation" and ensures that "all relevant voices are heard" (2004, p. 54). Qualitative approaches promote listening between researchers and the researched in order to get at "deeper, more genuine expressions of beliefs and values to foster a more accurate description of views held" and gather a more complex understanding of social life (p. 54). Additionally, qualitative approaches, because of their exploratory and theory-generating nature, tend to be oriented toward discovery of new phenomena and ways of understanding.

### Reasons for Mixing Methods from a Qualitative Approach

Qualitative researchers pursue a mixed methods design for a diverse range of reasons. Qualitative approaches typically employ a mixed methods design in which qualitative methods are primary or central to the research design. In discussing the motivations for using a mixed methods approach, we use the capitalized term "QUAL" to denote the dominance of the qualitative component of a study in a qualitative approach to mixed methods research design; the lowercased term "quan" is used to indicate the auxiliary role of the quantitative component in the figures on mixed methods designs shown throughout this chapter. Mixed methods designs also take into account whether or not the two studies are mixed sequentially (one, then the other) or concurrently (at the same time). There is also the issue of at what point(s) in the research projects the two studies are interacting with one another (at the data collection stage? data analysis and interpretation stage? both? neither?).

Researchers utilizing a qualitative approach might find some of the following mixed methods designs useful for their research projects for the reasons given after each example:

■ The researcher uses a quantitative study first with the goal of obtaining a *representative qualitative sample* for the purpose of enhancing his or her qualitative findings.

Conducting a quantitative demographic survey on a random sample of the researcher's target population first, followed by a qualitative study, enables the researcher to select a qualitative subsample from this population that is representative of the target population.

■ The researcher uses a quantitative study first to enhance the generalizability of a qualitative study.

The researcher uses findings from the quantitative study to select a qualitative sample that is reflective of the wider population in order to more readily generalize from in-depth research findings. This is especially the case when the researcher samples directly from the quantitative sample; in this way both studies are directly linked.

■ The qualitative researcher employs a quantitative method first in order to cast a wider net, with the goal of identifying a specific population of interest that may be hard to locate (*purposive sampling*).

For example, the researcher is interested in the lived experiences of HIV-positive males and finds it difficult to secure a large enough sample to interview. By first conducting a general health survey, a researcher might be able to locate a subsample for a follow-up set of intensive qualitative interviews, which in fact is the main motivation for conducting the survey.

■ Using a quantitative study first may help qualitative researchers define a population of interest based on specific research findings gathered from the quantitative study.

Suppose I am conducting a general social survey of caregivers' attitudes toward the elderly population. As a result of the findings from the quantitative study, I note the high degree of caregiver stereotyping of the elderly population, especially with regard to issues of race and gender. I may decide on the basis of these findings to conduct an in-depth study to explore caregiver's stereotypical attitudes by focusing specifically on caregivers employed in nursing homes. My focus of qualitative inquiry is sparked directly from the survey's findings.

- The researcher conducts a quantitative study first in order to examine its results as a way of generating new research questions that can be addressed in a follow-up qualitative study.

Mixed methods can assist qualitative researchers in identifying specific topical issues and concerns they wish to explore qualitatively. Here, the quantitative component serves to initiate or spark new hypotheses or research questions that qualitative researchers can pursue in depth. In addition, qualitative research can draw on quantitative findings to explore in more detail issues and discrepancies the researchers may find of interest to explore.

- Conducting a quantitative study first can provide options for enhancing the validity and reliability of qualitative findings, as well as for exploring contradictory results found between the quantitative and qualitative studies.

By linking the qualitative with the quantitative at the data-gathering stage (i.e., the researcher draws a qualitative sample directly from the quantitative sample first collected), the researcher is given the possibility of assessing the validity and reliability of her or his qualitative findings. For example, those qualitative researchers who ask similar questions in both the quantitative and qualitative studies have an opportunity to grapple with issues of reliability, validity, and contradiction of research findings by ascertaining (1) the extent to which research findings from similar questions yield similar responses (reliability) and (2) the extent to which their responses appear to get at the same underlying issues, such that there is general agreement in their responses (triangulation with the goal of increasing the validity of a study).

In addition, a qualitative researcher may decide to first conduct a sequential mixed methods design with the main qualitative study first and then seek to follow up with a quantitative study (QUAL $\rightarrow$ quan), as in the following example:

- The researcher uses a quantitative study to test the validity of qualitative findings on a wider population.

Findings from a qualitative study can be tested using a quantitative method. The researcher is interested in ascertaining whether the qualitative findings are applicable to a larger quantitative sample. This allows the researcher to generalize his or her qualitative results on a wider population.

A qualitative approach to mixed methods research may also employ both qualitative and quantitative studies concurrently for some of the following reasons:

- To gain a more robust understanding of qualitative results by integrating quantitative findings

- To triangulate the research findings

- To explore divergent or disparate findings

Quantitative data that are gathered may answer a different question, but at the data analysis stage, the findings from both these studies are in conversation with one another and appear to weave a richer and more complex story. Researchers may juxtapose the findings from each study and can interrogate the findings from one study to help understand the findings from the other. Sometimes the goal is to triangulate research findings; that is, researchers look at the extent to which results found using one method agree with the results found using another method (convergence). The goal here is to use mixed methods as a way to validate the research findings. Researchers can use a mixed methods design to explore the range of disparate findings they may discover in their mixed methods results in order to generate new questions and can explore these differences in order to gain a more complex understanding of their research problems. It is important to note that the researcher may weigh both studies equally depending on the research problem; in this case, the mixed methods design scenario is QUAL + QUAN.

## A Qualitative Approach to Mixed Methods Research Design

I inductively derived a set of mixed methods design "templates" that are based on the preceding reasons that qualitatively driven researchers might want to use mixed methods. These templates, however, do not cover the variety of all reasons or the range of all mixed methods designs that one might select from. These templates should be thought of as working models of mixed methods designs that can be tweaked, added to, or deleted, depending on the particular research problem or set of problems that emerge during the course of the research project. I advocate this iterative approach to mixed methods design given that the nature of a qualitative approach to research is often subject to change as the research project proceeds and alters its course in response to new research findings, which in turn may prompt new research questions along the way.

### Some Inductively Generated Mixed Methods Templates

In the following section, I depict examples of both parallel mixed methods designs and sequential mixed methods designs that a qualitative approach to research might find useful. The important thing to note is that all these designs are in the service of answering a qualitative research question.

#### Parallel Mixed Methods Design

Parallel mixed methods designs consist of the concurrent mixing of qualitative and quantitative methods carried out as separate studies within the same research project, with the qualitative component taking a more dominant role. In one particular instance, the qualitative researcher may be motivated to design a parallel research project in order to gather some descriptive quantitative information, such as demographic statistics of the population that he or she studies, in order to place the findings from the qualitative study into a larger context (see Figure 3.1).

If a researcher who favors qualitative data uses a parallel mixed methods design, he or she tends not to engage directly with the quantitative data; the quantitative component is often used to "window dress" a primarily qualitative approach to a project. In some instances, the quantitative data are embedded in the qualitative data, signifying their secondary role. The synergy between the two datasets is not usually present. Data are not mixed at any stage of the research process, except perhaps at the writing stage, in which quantitative methods are mentioned as a backdrop to the dominant qualitative findings.

Although this design presents limited opportunities for integration at data analysis and interpretation points in the research process,

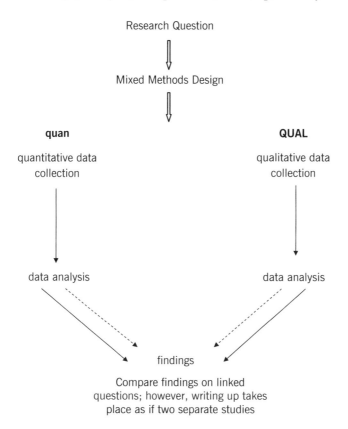

**FIGURE 3.1.** Parallel mixed methods design. Sometimes the quantitative study (quan) is "nested" within the qualitative study (QUAL). The dashed line represents a missed opportunity to compare findings from both studies; in a parallel study, this is not always done. The solid line, however, represents a comparison of the findings (the opportunity taken). The quantitative component may also take on an equivalent importance (QUAN), depending on the research problem.

a parallel design may still offer the researcher some opportunities for more direct engagement of datasets by having the researcher engage in reflexivity regarding how her or his quantitative findings may raise new questions that are connected in some substantive way to the research problem rather than using the quantitative data atheoretically. For instance, the researcher might seek out points of connection, guided by her or his original research question, at both the data analysis and data interpretation stages, by consciously comparing and contrasting the research findings from both datasets. More often than not, however, the nonconnection of these different data points usually serves to underscore the divide between the two methods, not their potential synergistic connection.

A parallel design is currently one of the most common forms of mixed methods designs used in quantitative approaches to triangulate, or corroborate, a specific research finding (Bryman, 2008, p. 93). These researchers use a qualitative study to buttress the results of their more dominant quantitative method. Some researchers taking a qualitative approach may use a parallel design for triangulating their qualitative data with the quantitative data to corroborate their predominately qualitative findings. It is also important to note that researchers who take a qualitative approach that begins with the goal of triangulation are much more open to disparate findings that may result from their attempts at triangulation. Rather than dismissing their quantitative findings when they contradict the qualitative results, these research-ers are open to using them as an opportunity to rethink their overall research objectives, seeing them as potentially important insights into their primarily qualitative studies.

A parallel design is also used for those research projects with both dominant qualitative and dominant quantitative components, although in this instance they address different aspects of a larger research prob-lem. It is most likely that researchers from each component of the study are from different disciplines that hold different *methodological perspec-tives* regarding the nature of the social world. This is a more collabora-tive version of a parallel design that may open more opportunities for research findings from each component to connect, perhaps promot-ing a cross-fertilization of ideas. However, the extent to which the differ-ent components of the project become integrated may depend on how well the research question(s) posed from this parallel design contains aspects relatable to both perspectives. For example, if the research ques-tion calls for explicitly linking both macro and micro levels of under-standing, it becomes analytically feasible to combine and connect the findings from both studies. However, this may not be enough to pro-mote the integration of findings. There may be certain structural issues that stem from working on a cross-disciplinary or interdisciplinary team project that have not been thought through; for example, issues such as who decides how the study will be integrated and reported.

Parallel designs hold much promise for qualitative and quantita-tive approaches to research. However, a recent study regarding how researchers practice and think about mixed methods research reveals that, with regard to parallel mixed methods designs, most mixed meth-ods researchers interviewed for this project did not integrate their mixed methods at any stage of the project. Their studies remained parallel but separate throughout the research process (Bryman, 2008, p. 98).

### Sequential Mixed Method Design

Qualitative approaches to research employ sequential mixed methods designs in which the quantitative study (quan) is in the service of the more dominant qualitative (QUAL) one. The studies are sequential in that one study follows and builds on the next (see Figure 3.2).

In a *sequential exploratory mixed methods design*, the qualitative component is primary and is used to generate theory or specific theoretical constructs. The quantitative component is used in the service of the qualitative in that it "tests out" ideas generated from the qualitative component. The model itself is an iterative design in which theory generated from the qualitative component is tested out on a representative population, findings are compared, and then, if needed, the theory is revised and tested out again in an ongoing process of theory generation and testing in a series of "wave" studies (see Figure 3.3).

Sometimes a researcher taking a qualitative approach uses a sequential design in order to find out more about his or her target sample or to obtain a more representative sample for further in-depth investigation of the research problem. In this case, the sequential study is not

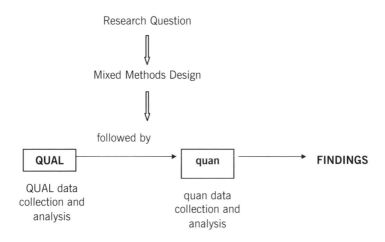

**FIGURE 3.2.** QUAL → quan sequential exploratory design. Quantitative data results assist in the interpretation of qualitative findings: (1) testing aspects of an emergent theory, (2) generalizing qualitative findings to different samples, and (3) validating a specific set of survey items (adapted from Creswell, 2003).

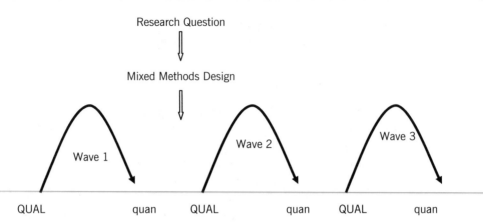

**FIGURE 3.3.** Integrating methods in a sequential exploratory design (one method "talks" to the other). This is the continual, iterative theory-generation and testing model over time. This wave study could be replicated beginning with the quantitative study leading the wave, but a qualitatively driven researcher would want to start with theory generation (QUAL) in this wave model.

done for exploratory but for data gathering purposes, with the goal of generalizing and validating the qualitative analysis and interpretation. Figure 3.4 is an "explanatory" sequential mixed methods design.

Researchers can also integrate the data from both studies in this explanatory mixed methods design at the data interpretation stage by allowing for the comparison of research findings, especially if the two studies have utilized similar questions of interest to the research question. This would serve to increase the validity of the qualitative results and potentially provide a more complex understanding of qualitative results when an apparent contradiction exists.

## A Qualitative Approach to Analysis and Interpretation of Mixed Methods Research

In this section, we examine the problems of mixing methods across a research project and why most mixed methods designs often fail to achieve the potential synergy that resides in employing mixed methods research. We do so by examining some of the particular barriers to mixing methods at the point of analysis and interpretation of data. We specifically pinpoint those issues that researchers taking a qualitative approach face in analyzing and interpreting a mixed methods

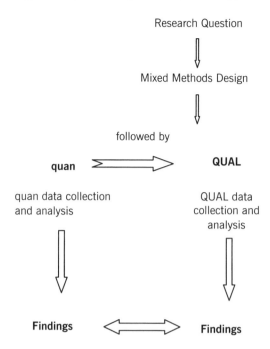

**FIGURE 3.4.** quan → QUAL sequential explanatory design. Findings from each study may be compared and contrasted with the goals of (1) generalizing qualitative findings to different samples and (2) validating and/or comparing findings from similar questions asked in quan.

project and present some general guidelines for mixing of methods at both these stages. In our view, analysis and interpretation are separate stages of the research process, with analysis involving the deconstruction of data into various component parts and interpretation involving meaning making and theory building. Finally, we address the role of computer-assisted qualitative data analysis software (CAQDAS) in the analysis and interpretation of data gathered from a mixed methods project. I provide some specific examples of how this can be done in Appendices 3.1 and 3.2 at the end of this chapter.

### Mixing Methodologies in the Analysis and Interpretation of Mixed Methods Data

These mixed methods design templates suggest the ways in which researchers who take a qualitative approach may find points of connection to quantitative data throughout their research inquiry. Promoting a fuller integration of mixed methods designs, however, may require that the researcher move toward a more methodologically mixed set of research questions that call for a crossing of methodological boundaries. Mixing methodologies and methods does not necessarily make for a more robust or synergistic study; often a researcher can best address an issue or problem from one methodological approach.

One of the most important factors in whether or not mixed methods designs are integrated at the analysis and interpretation stage is *awareness* on the part of the researchers of their own paradigmatic or methodological position. Giddings and Grant (2007) note that without this awareness one of the two methods may be included in a superficial manner, or, in some cases, the findings from one may be rejected if they do not agree with other research results (p. 58).

Researchers are often housed in specific disciplines, which, in turn, are rooted in particular research methodologies; these methodologies, as I mentioned in Chapter 1, have their own assumptions about the nature of reality, as well as favored methods that are perceived as foundational to their research approach. So, for example, researchers working from a positivistic paradigm, whose methodology assumes a unified social reality, may feel more comfortable using quantitative methods whose goals are to test out hypotheses and to make generalizations about this reality.

An understanding and appreciation of the potential contributions that different methodological viewpoints bring to a mixed methods study may then be necessary for deeper integration of mixed methods designs; otherwise, difference is treated as addition or even omission but not as integration. For example, a positivist researcher may juxtapose the qualitative component of his or her research project with the quantitative component with little interaction between the two methods, in effect running parallel qualitative and quantitative components. Such work remains "unmixed," with perhaps more loyalty given to the methodology the researcher is most comfortable with, leaving methodological boundaries unchallenged.

### The Mixed Methodological Standpoint

Adopting a multimethodological perspective, then, is often a process in which one becomes both an insider and an outsider, taking on a multitude of different standpoints and negotiating these identities simultaneously. This was aptly expressed by Trinh T. Minh-ha's (1992) concept of multiple subjectivities:

Working right at the limits of several categories and approaches means that one is neither entirely inside or outside. One has to push one's work as far as one can go: to the borderlines, where one never stops walking on the edges, incurring constantly the risk of falling off one side or the other side of the limit while undoing, redoing, modifying this limit. (Minh-ha, 1992, p. 218)

Working from mixed methodological standpoints requires a keen sense of interdisciplinarity. Klein's (1990) research on successful inter-disciplinary scholars applies to those who are successful in working across diverse methodologies and who require "reliability, flexibility, patience, resilience, sensitivity to others, risk-taking, a thick skin, and a preference for diversity and new social roles" (p. 183). Good communication skills among colleagues from different points of view, noted Klein, is a necessity, and the wider the gap between standpoints, the larger the number of methodologies involved and the higher the potential for communication gaps (p. 183). For now, we offer some initial guidelines for a qualitative approach to a mixed methods project at different stages in the research process that flow from our examination of the templates discussed earlier (see Figure 3.5).

Figure 3.5 presents the range of decision steps researchers may confront throughout their mixed methods research undertaking. This mixed methods model is somewhat simplified, because several iterations of the model may develop as researchers gather data, analyze and interpret them, and find that they need to collect additional data using more than one additional method. The model we provide is theory and question driven, which is central to a mixed methods design. Several outside factors such as stakeholder values, the literature review, and one's disciplinary structure may also affect the researcher's decision-making process along the way. Figure 3.5 also presents a series of guideposts that researchers might reflect on as their mixed methods project progresses. Very often mixed methods projects integrate methods at the analysis, interpretation, and writing stages of the project. The following are additional guidelines.

## Guidelines for Mixing Methods at the Data Analysis and Interpretation Stage

Here we outline some guidelines for analysis and interpretation to consider at the outset of your mixed methods research project.

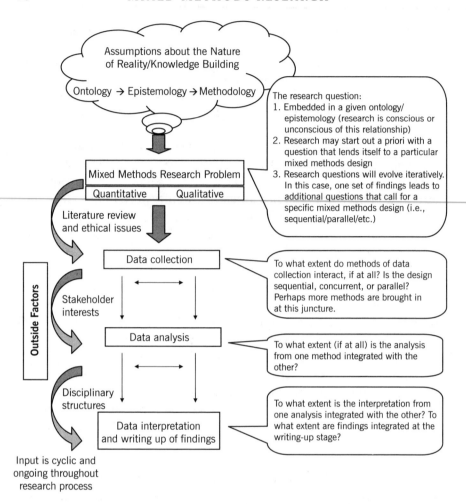

**FIGURE 3.5.** The mixed method process: Theory and praxis.

■ The findings of both methods should be thoroughly addressed and integrated if possible. Researchers should neither subsume the results of one method under the findings of the more dominant method nor neglect the results altogether.

■ Researchers should be committed to integrating their research findings from both methods. In other words, the findings from both methods should be in conversation with one another.

- Data analysis and data interpretation in a mixed methods design may be more successfully integrated in an interdisciplinary project, in which researchers are trained in a variety of methods.

- There is the risk that the findings from one method are privileged over the other, creating a lack of real integration in the interpretation. This will be overcome with reflexivity and experience in using both methods.

We turn now to a more in-depth look at some specific approaches to mixed methods analysis and interpretation that can apply to a range of mixed methods research approaches, although this discussion centers on qualitative approaches to mixed methods.

### Analysis and Interpretation of Qualitative Approaches to Mixed Methods Data

In their book *On Writing Qualitative Research: Living by Words* (1999), Ely, Vinz, Anzul, and Downing defined qualitative analysis as the "separating of material (text) into its constituent elements or thinking units" (p. 162) and interpretation as the process of "drawing meaning from the analyzed data and attempting to see these in some larger [theoretical] context" (p. 160). Although analysis and interpretation are separate processes, they are intertwined, as Ely et al. (1999) noted: "The interweaving of data collection and analysis is highly transactional, each activity shedding new light on and enriching the other. The choice of foci for close observation in the field is very much a part of the analytic process" (p. 165).

You need to consider some general points as you contemplate integrating qualitative and quantitative research findings at the data analysis and interpretation stage. First, skill level has a large bearing on integrating your data. When a researcher using mixed methods is poorly trained in one of the data analysis methods, he or she may tend to subsume or give less weight to the less understood method than to the more familiar method at the data analysis stage, potentially resulting in a favoring of one type of findings over another.

Integrating the analysis and interpretation of research results becomes more complex when two or more theoretical frameworks are used, each of which asks different questions with perhaps different findings. In this case, the researcher must assess how to integrate these findings into the understanding of the research problem(s), especially if the findings do not agree with each other. This type of situation becomes problematic if the researcher tries to discount or downplay the findings from one method in favor of the other or decides instead to report each of the findings without talking about how they are related—a sort of parallel presentation of research findings for each study with a separate interpretation. The following section provides information on specific analytical tools for mixing methods at the data analysis and data interpretation stages.

### Analyzing Mixed Methods Using Computer-Assisted Qualitative Data Analysis Software

The advent of new computer-based technologies has also prompted an increased interest in combining a variety of methods. Computer-assisted software programs for analyzing qualitative data are beginning to seek ways to incorporate and integrate quantitative data into their programs. The introduction of CAQDAS has enabled researchers to begin to transform qualitative and quantitative data to suit their methodological purposes (see Fielding & Lee, 1998a; Hesse-Biber & Dupuis, 1995; Hesse-Biber, Dupuis, & Kinder, 1991).

Some qualitative software programs are designed so that the researcher may import quantitative data, such as data gathered from a survey, into the computer software program, making it possible for the researcher to work with both the qualitative and quantitative databases at the same time. They also are useful for analyzing large sets of data that do not lend themselves to hand coding.

With growing technological advancements in qualitative data analysis programs, researchers are increasingly able to utilize new methods to develop theories and test them on qualitative materials. Knowledge-based systems, such as artificial intelligence programs, are particularly useful. One such program, HyperRESEARCH, a CAQDAS program, uses a "hypothesis tester" to develop "if–then" propositions that allow a researcher to expand or develop his or her hypotheses. HyperRESEARCH creates and analyzes relationships between coded text segments using production rules, and this helps to generate and test the proposed hypotheses (Hesse-Biber & Dupuis, 1995). Another, similar program, ETHNO (Heise, 1991; Heise & Lewis, 1988), is a software program that performs an event structure analysis, examining the timing of specific events. ETHNO evaluates the logical temporal sequence of relationships between events by looking at causal narratives within data.[2]

## CAQDAS Techniques for Transforming Data: Quantizing and Qualitizing

CAQDAS programs allow researchers to group their qualitative (textual) data, such as interview material, into "variable-like" categories. *Quantizing* occurs when qualitative *codes* (labels given to segments of data from texts that have been transcribed from interviews or other narrative sources, such as magazines or newspapers) are transformed into quantitative variables. Quantizing opens up the possibility of applying statistical techniques to material that was once qualitative. Miles and Huberman (1994) were the first researchers to use the term "quantizing" (see also Sandelowski, 2000b; Sandelowski et al., 2009).

*Qualitizing,* on the other hand, refers to the transformation of quantitative data into qualitative data. This transformation process was first developed by Tashakorri and Teddlie (1998) and is not often addressed in the mixed methods literature (see Tashakkori & Teddlie, 1998; also Sandelowski, 2000a, pp. 253–254). One might think of this process as making quantitative data more qualitative by taking numerical data from individual case studies—for example, a respondent's score on an eating disorder test—and transforming them into ordinal-level data categories (high, medium, and low) for each case in the study. Qualitizing often uses empirically grounded information provided by the qualitative component of the mixed methods study as well as the research literature to decide how to determine what the cutoff points will be for each of the categories. In a sense, the research is using what might be termed "fuzzy" categorizing—not just depending on the quantitative scoring index to determine what should be considered "high," "medium," or "low" but also using empirically grounded information from both the qualitative component of the mixed methods project and the literature (see Ragin, 2000).[3] Qualitized quantitative data can be integrated with qualitative data and provide the researcher with a set of qualitized categories with which to sort through all the data, and I provide an example of this in Appendix 3.2. For a diagram of qualitizing and quantizing, refer to Figure 3.6.

The ability to quantize qualitative data turns traditional positivist research on its head and allows the researcher to view patterns and numbers of qualitative data and to manipulate statistical techniques.

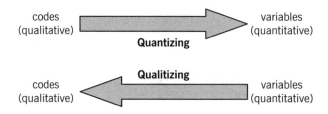

**FIGURE 3.6.** Data transformation: Qualitizing and quantizing.

A mixed data analysis design helps build a framework within which one can identify and understand variables derived from quantitative data. However, one must not ignore the issues that arise when utilizing quantizing or qualitizing techniques; the quantitative and qualitative analytical realms remain separate.

### A Cautionary Note on Using Computer Software Programs to Analyze Mixed Methods Data

The growing use of computer software programs as tools for mixed methods analysis and qualitative analysis in general raises a number of concerns regarding how data are analyzed and interpreted. These new techniques should be applied with caution and attention to relevant issues, conceptual (epistemological–methodological issues) and practical (e.g., choosing an appropriate statistical tool for analyzing qualitative variables and choosing how to interpret findings). Quantizing qualitative data into codes and then variables raises concerns for researchers, because it can conflict with important assumptions about how phenomena are measured. This becomes a particular concern especially when the data do not come from standardized question format but instead from nonstandardized qualitative instruments such as open-ended interviews or ethnographic field notes—a method that is not designed to capture discrete and consistent responses in a systematic manner, as in a survey.

Not all would respond similarly to these criticisms. One counterargument points to the issue that many of those interviewed, when given the opportunity to talk about their lives, will in fact discuss those issues they feel are most salient in their lives; therefore, the interview may not need to be standardized because the interviewee's attention would most likely direct itself toward what they consider to be the most important set of "codes" (Hesse-Biber & Carter, 2004). Concern also abounds over the type of analysis that should be applied to data that have been quantized and whether the analysis should be limited to standard procedures (i.e., statistical measures of the relationships between variables) or extended to complex statistical procedures (e.g., performing a log-linear analysis).

In order to address these issues, researchers are advised to be constantly aware of the most basic goals of their mixed methods projects, and the need to practice reflexivity, remaining aware of their epistemological positions. It is important to remember that these concerns may not be relevant to every type of research study and that the issues must be examined on a case-by-case basis. If a qualitative researcher is well trained in quantitative research methods, he or she may be open to using quantized variables as an important heuristic device that reveals different patterns and links between data. Utilizing the method of quantizing variables can help pinpoint codes and create more specific survey questions, for example. Quantification is not the end point but rather "a means of making available techniques which add power and sensitivity to individual judgment when one attempts to detect and describe patterning in a set of observations" (Weinstein & Tamur, 1978, p. 140, quoted in Miles & Huberman, 1994, p. 41).

Further concerns have been raised about the use of computer software programs for analyzing data. Hesse-Biber (1995), for example, noted that one fear that critics express is that these programs will separate the qualitatively driven researcher from his or her creative process. Some researchers consider the experience of qualitative work to be akin to artistic work; "just as the artist prefers a brush or pencil and paper, so too do some qualitative researchers" (Hesse-Biber, 1995, p. 27). These critics view the use of computer technology as incompatible with the intuitive and creative elements of qualitative research work. Another concern critics express is that the ability of CAQDAS programs to qualitize and quantize data from mixed methods studies blurs the distinction between what is quantitative and what is qualitative data analysis. There is especially a fear that qualitative work will be reduced to quantitative, because by using CAQDAS qualitative researchers can generate counts of the occurrences of their coded categories and transport them to a matrix for statistical analysis. Additionally, critics also fear that the very structure of software programs themselves may serve to dictate what types of research questions are asked and how specific data analysis procedures will be performed.

Computer software programs, then, promise to revolutionize analysis of mixed methods data, but they hold some peril, especially for a qualitative analysis approach. Those who employ these programs need to assess their strengths and limitations and the further implications of using them to analyze their data.

After data analysis and interpretation of mixed methods results, the researcher takes this new information and begins the writing-up process. We are reminded of Denzin's comments that "writing is not an innocent practice" but a method that can help us to interpret and change the world (2001, p. ix).

## Writing Up Mixed Methods Projects

The mixed methods literature has not addressed the important issue of writing up the results of this type of study. Part of this may stem from the fact that publishing outlets for mixed methods research are somewhat limited, and, as Julia Brannen noted, "academic journals tend to be organised around disciplines and may favour particular types of research. Moreover different types of data analyses may sit awkwardly together on the published page and may require rather a lot of space to justify their validity and credibility" (Brannen, 2005, p. 26).

As a result of this publishing barrier, Brannen noted that mixed methods researchers tend to prioritize in their write-ups either the qualitative or quantitative components of their studies, depending on which method is privileged by a given journal. In addition, the structure of journal articles may limit the space allotted to reporting of research findings, and this in turn may cause researchers to truncate their reporting of results. The page limits of many journal articles, as well as the page limits and/or templates of grant applications, may make it difficult for researchers to explain their mixed methods designs and findings in only several paragraphs. Additionally, journal reviewers may not be familiar with mixed methods research. These publishing constraints limit the reporting of the mixed methods findings. Bryman (2006) conducted a content analysis of 232 mixed methods articles from 1994 to 2003. He found that only 18% of these articles integrated the qualitative and quantitative components of the research project.

If a researcher decides to write up her or his research findings, few exemplary mixed methods projects exist that the researcher can use as a template. Bryman (2007a) wrote:

> insufficient attention has been paid to the writing up of mixed methods findings and in particular to the ways in which such findings can

be integrated. Indeed, it could be argued that there is still considerable uncertainty concerning what it means to integrate findings in mixed methods research. The relative absence of well-known exemplars of mixed methods research makes this exercise particularly difficult, as it means that scholars have few guidelines upon which to draw when writing up their findings. (Bryman, 2007a, p. 21)

Mixed methods researchers who work in multidisciplinary or interdisciplinary team projects may be working in a parallel manner (i.e., they have a common research problem, but they approach it separately from their particular ontology/epistemology) without considering points of convergence and divergence of their research findings. To work across disciplinary boundaries requires good communication and a thick skin. How are differing viewpoints addressed in the writing up of a project? Team building takes time, energy, and resources in order to sustain a project over time. There is also little discussion in the literature on what makes for a successful interdisciplinary or multidisciplinary mixed methods structure. (For an exception, see Simons [2007].)

In addition to these structural problems concerning mixed methods research project publication, researchers are advised to pay attention to style of writing and the notion of what counts as "evidence" in deciding how to report their findings. Epistemological assumptions also affect the researcher's choice of writing style, because any particular view comes embedded with a set of writing paradigms, and researchers must parse out their own underlying viewpoints before undertaking a mixed methods project write-up.

Researchers may try to achieve different goals in their research writing. As Carol Bailey (1996) stated, research writing either takes the shape of a "realist tale" or a "nonrealist tale" (p. 106). A realist tale follows the traditional writing style; the write-up is prepared for publication in a report, book, or journal and often assumes the role of being a "true" reflection of a single social reality, with the researcher's individual voice taking a back seat to the "disembodied voice of authority" (see also Hesse-Biber & Leavy, 2006e, p. 365). Realist tales seek to identify patterns of occurrence and behavior within a sample set, often testing out hypotheses and concentrating on concrete details (Bailey, 1996, p. 106).

On the other hand, a nonrealist tale, often a result of a qualitative research approach, is less rigid and more concerned with pushing the boundaries of traditional research writing. Bailey (1996) and Richardson (1994) both note that an important aspect of nonrealist tales is their attention to the voices of the respondents and to acknowledging the power dynamics inherent in researcher–researched relationships. This type of research writing acknowledges that multitudes of voices need to be examined but that even this does not provide a complete understanding of the social realities that are researched.

### To Integrate or Not to Integrate?

Given the comprehensive approach to mixed methods research that I advocate in this book, I view the writing process as tightly linked to the research question(s) of the study. The extent to which the findings of both methods are integrated and what the "best" mix should be is guided by the research problem at hand. The research problem should dictate how results and conclusions from both methods are written up; that is, whether researchers should write up results separately and then combine them into a general conclusion or whether they should integrate the results in an ongoing process (see Figure 3.7).

Practicing reflexivity is an important technique to utilize as you begin to write up your mixed methods research project. The following are some guidelines we might consider as we write up our research findings:

■ Know your own standpoint as a researcher. What particular biases do you bring to or impose on your research? This means reflecting on your own assumptions about the nature of the social world (questions about ontology and epistemology). Knowing your own standpoint will guide you in making decisions about how you want to present your work

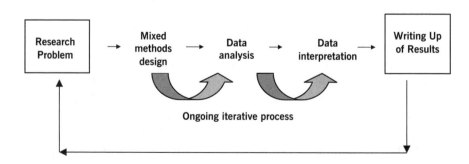

**FIGURE 3.7.** Writing up of mixed methods research results.

(i.e., as a realist tale or a nonrealist tale), which audiences you are most interested in reaching through your writing, and so forth.

■ Examine your analytic biases. Are you wedded to one type of methods practice? Do you feel open to working with different methods and writing up research findings from multiple methods?

■ Examine your methods skill level. Are you comfortable working with both qualitative and quantitative data? Are you knowledgeable about how you might integrate mixed methods data? Would you consider a team-based project for which you bring in others whose skills you need to complete this project?

■ If you are working with a research team, has your research team reflected together on how research findings will or will not be integrated? Remember that it will take social skills and time for research teams, especially those who hold different assumptions about the nature of the social world, to work together.

■ To what extent are you attentive to difference in your research findings? To what extent have you focused on issues of race, class, gender, and so on?

■ How will you deal with divergent findings? Within a mixed methods project, you may come up with a range of disparate findings. How open are you to disparate findings in your data?

The next section explores the critical issues of validity and reliability in qualitative approaches to mixed methods research.

## Validity and Reliability in Mixed Methods Research[4]

Positivism places a high premium on "objectivity" in the research process, which affects the research methods that are used in a project. An important component in the validity of a positivistic study is its measures. Validity asks: Do the instruments measure the phenomenon that they are supposed to? Reliability asks: If I use the same measure today and repeat it again on the same population shortly thereafter, will I obtain the same results?

The positivist tradition's view of social reality as "knowable," then, is tied to a view of classic validity strictly in terms of measurement.

Kvale (1996) noted that "in a positivist philosophy, knowledge became a reflection of reality: There is only one correct view of the independent external world, and there is ideally a one-to-one correspondence between elements in the real world and our knowledge of this world" (p. 239).

Issues of validity and reliability are different in qualitative research approaches. A primary assumption of qualitative approaches, for the most part, is that social reality is socially constructed. Employing a definition of validity as "correspondence with the objective world" is not realistic. Kvale's (1996) alternate definition of validity is that "validity is ascertained by examining the sources of invalidity. The stronger the falsification attempts a proposition has survived, the more valid, the trustworthier the knowledge" (Kvale, 1996, p. 241). In this light, validity takes the form of looking at mixed methods findings and interrogating them: What is not there? What frame or subjective experiences negate that finding? (Kvale, 1996).

### Mixed Methods and Issues of Validity

Within the mixed methods field, discussions of validity and reliability often take the form of a *methods-centric discussion* regarding the mismatch of mixed methods design elements. A cursory examination of some mixed methods textbooks and articles finds guidelines for validity that mostly focus on the "correctness" of design procedures. For example, the types of questions these textbooks pose are the following:

> Does the research use both qualitative and quantitative data, and, if so, are they mixed?
>
> Is the correct type of terminology employed?
>
> Does the study give a good reason for using mixed methods?
>
> Does the study state clearly that its purpose was to mix methods?
>
> Does the study clearly state the mixed methods steps involved in collecting and analyzing the data?

We can see from the preceding questions that the validation process centers on having the correct mixed methods design and that validation requires having the right *methods elements*. The emphasis on validation does not center on whether or not the research findings from the study are valid. The research question enters the discussion of validity as disembodied from the method. The research question enters a discussion of validity only as part of a two-part checklist:

- To make sure the research question is asked
- To make sure that there is a rationale for explaining the reasons that the researcher chose a particular mixed methods design

What is missing from the discussion of mixed methods validity is how well the problem and method are *linked*; namely, whether the method provides a "goodness of fit" to answer the original problem and question(s). This is critical in assessing the validity of any study, but in particular a mixed methods study, given the complexity of designs that one might select from and the already "methods-centric" nature of the field. A second set of questions regarding validity in a mixed methods study is:

- How well do the researcher's findings fit the problem? In other words, did her or his findings capture the issue (problem) at hand?
- How well does the researcher answer her or his research question(s)?
- Did the research capture an understanding of the issue?

### Assessing Validity in a Qualitative Approach to Mixed Methods

Before the validity of a study can be assessed, you need to go back to your research problem statement to ascertain the type of validation procedure you should consider (see also Kvale, 1996, p. 243). There may, in fact, be multiple research questions, and this may be particularly true in a mixed methods design (more so when the researcher is mixing methodologies). Some research questions may require a more quantitative validation procedure, whereas others may rely on a qualitative assessment of validation that relies, for example, on the "trustworthiness" of the data at hand. Some mixed methods studies may require a *mixed process of validation*, using qualitative and quantitative approaches to validation.

Another important aspect of validity is an assessment of how well researchers have done in generating theoretical understanding of the given problems they address in their mixed methods studies (Kvale,

1996, p. 244). Are researchers convincing about what they have to say? Are they able to present a "goodness of fit" between their theoretical ideas and the final story (data analysis and findings)? Do the data fit the researcher's theoretical frame? Does the story seem to capture an important aspect of knowledge building? Do the results provide a better understanding of the problem? Has something important been left out?

Kvale (1996) suggested three criteria of validation for any given qualitative study that can also apply to a qualitative approach to mixed methods: (1) validity as the quality of craftsmanship, (2) validity as communication, and (3) pragmatic validity as action (p. 241). Whereas validity as craftsmanship involves how well the different pieces of your research fit together and correspond with the research question posed, validity as communication and pragmatic validity concern how well your research translates to and finds legitimacy in the community of experts in your field and the degree to which your research is able to have a practical impact in the wider world. Let's look at each of these criteria for assessing validity in more detail.

## Validity as a Quality of Craftsmanship

Validity as craftsmanship implies that an individual assessing this research project feels that the research has a high degree of credibility, what Kvale termed "moral integrity" (Kvale, 1996, p. 241). This integrity and credibility are confirmed as the result of examining the researcher's actions throughout the research process. How careful has the researcher been in double checking his or her findings? Does he or she go back, for example, to the original data when a question of an inconsistency arises in the reported results? Has the researcher left what you feel are important questions or concerns unanswered? Has the researcher been reflexive about how his or her own point of view might have compromised the findings? These types of validity checks on a study also affect its degree of reliability. Within these questions is also an assessment of how well the parts of a study work together and whether or not there are built-in cross-checks. Having these cross-checks in place raises the possibility of increasing the reliability of the mixed methods study. By following up at specific points in the research process, we create a built-in mechanism for catching some of those errors that may lead to a breakdown of research operations and make a study less reliable and valid.

One interesting thing to note in this regard is the relationship between validity and reliability, especially within a mixed methods study. The more a researcher seeks to get at a given social problem, the more he or she may, in fact, increase the validity of a study; that is, in the case of a qualitative approach, he or she may enhance understanding. However, as layers that are more subjective are uncovered through this process, the reliability of the study begins to decrease as it becomes more difficult to replicate results. An example to illustrate the tension between validity and reliability comes from attempts of social researchers to measure a respondent's age. You might think that the way to get the most accurate (valid) measure of someone's age is to ask him or her how old he or she is. However, if you try to do so on a questionnaire by asking, "What is your age?" the answers may not be as valid as if respondents were asked to select an age category from a set of age intervals, for example, 15–20 years of age and so on. Although the exact-age question in theory has high validity, asking this exact-age question on a survey negatively influences its reliability. Reliability decreases because many respondents may decide to give you their age on their next birthdays; some may feel the question is too personal and do not want to reveal their exact age; and so on. Furthermore, if you repeat the exact-age question the next day to the same respondent, you may not necessarily get the same answer as you did the day before, also affecting the reliability of this measure. In order to negotiate the tension between validity and reliability, a researcher may often trade off a little validity (exact-age question) for some reliability (using an interval-age question instead).

The idea of even entertaining a concept of reliability in general when applied to qualitative approaches to mixed methods study design almost seems like an oxymoron, because an important goal of qualitative research is to get at multiple understandings. Even if one replicates this type of design the next day and gets a different answer, it does not necessarily mean the mixed methods study was not reliable. Instead, what it may mean is that the researcher uncovered a new layer of meaning to the problem.

The process of validation also investigates what is "under the hood" of any given mixed methods study—looking at methods procedures, both qualitative and quantitative, not just issues regarding design construction. Validation asks such questions as, Does the research contain both a quantitative and a qualitative component? Is the terminology correct? Researchers should be aware of how well they perform their analysis of each dataset with regard to the specific research question it is supposed to be investigating. So, for instance, check to make sure that a sample selection matches the primary research questions. Another important aspect of checking data for validity in the qualitative portion of a study is performing what is called a "negative case analysis." This process involves checking for *negative cases*, which are the results that do not seem to fit the final analysis (Glaser & Strauss, 1967). If a researcher comes up with an idea or a key relationship in the data, he or she must go out of his or her way to look for negative instances in which the relationship does not hold up in the data and then try to adjust the theory in order to explain the apparent contradiction. Very often, this is done as an ongoing procedure throughout one's study, especially if one is using a more grounded theory approach to research.

Another important type of validity check involves exploring and entertaining alternative theoretical explanations for findings. Researchers must critically examine their own findings, mentioning the strengths and weaknesses of their arguments and offering alternative explanations for the research results (Kvale, 1996, p. 242).

The next two types of validity have to do with the review process, looking at whether the study makes sense to consumers of this research, experts in the field as well as the wider research community.

## Communicative Validity

Another form of validation is communicative validity. At this stage those who might be thought of as experts regarding the particular research problem get together to evaluate, debate, and dialogue about the claims or findings of the research, moving toward the idea of more "intersubjectivity," or shared consensus on its meaning. Communication brings validity in that, although not all the experts will agree, there is a sense that all viewpoints on this topic are heard and shared and that there is room to perhaps resolve disagreements (Kvale, 1996, pp. 244–245). Although this sounds good in theory, the practice of determining who is an "expert" can be tricky, and it could be that the criteria used to select experts are themselves fraught with power dynamics that might serve to shut out some differing points of view or those whose opinions may serve to construct a carefully crafted consensus.

## Pragmatic Validity

Whereas communicative validity reaches an understanding concerning knowledge claims within the wider research community and beyond, pragmatic validity examines the extent to which research findings affect both those studied and the wider context within which the study was conducted. Depending on the type of study conducted and the findings, one would expect to look for certain "action" outcomes. For example, suppose I am interested in the validity of a questionnaire I filled out on a dating website that promises to match my profile with that of a compatible person. A pragmatic validity check would consist of my personal assessment of the veracity of the profile tested against whether or not I found it useful by asking: Did the profile match me with someone I felt compatible with? Kvale (1996) noted:

> Pragmatic validation raises the issue of power and truth in social research: Where is the power to decide what the desired results of a study will be, or the direction of change; what values are to constitute the basis for action? And, more generally, where is the power to decide what kinds of truth seeking are to be pursued, what research questions are worth funding? (p. 251)

### Assessing Validity and Reliability for Mixed Methods Research Using a Mixed Evaluation Approach

Just what the evaluation criteria for validity and reliability of mixed methods designs should be is dependent on the problem–methods linkage of a given mixed methods study. As Maxwell (1992) noted early on:

> a method by itself is neither valid nor invalid: methods can produce valid data or accounts in some circumstances and invalid ones in others. Validity is not an inherent property of a particular method, but pertains to the data, accounts or conclusions reached by using that method in a particular context for a particular purpose. (p. 284)

A more qualitative approach might call for a method of assessing validity and reliability that is less quantifiable (i.e., validity or reliability coefficients would not be an appropriate assessment of validity). Instead, the means of ensuring validity and reliability will involve maintaining an ongoing set of *researcher dialogues* across the research process between the researcher and the stakeholders in any given mixed methods study, regarding their perceptions of the fit between the problem and the method. The use of subjective measures of validity and reliability, as we have outlined here, may be the most appropriate way to evaluate mixed methods research projects taking a qualitative approach. However, mixed methods designs may ultimately call for researchers to move across a continuum of quantitative and qualitative measures of validation procedures, depending on the uniqueness of the particular problem–design nexus of any given mixed methods study. This is particularly the case when researchers mix methodologies as well as methods.

The next chapters examine how researchers with differing theoretical approaches (i.e., interpretative, feminist, and postmodern) use mixed methods. We highlight the ways in which these alternative theoretical perspectives inform the way mixed methods research is currently practiced and what the points of tension and agreement are between these alternative points of view on the social reality. We address the researchers who define themselves as working from one or several of these approaches and consider what type of questions within each of these approaches lend themselves to the pursuit of a mixed methods design.

---

### APPENDIX 3.1. Quantizing Qualitative Data[5]

There are some simple ways in which qualitative data can be turned into numbers (quantized) using the following quantitative techniques. We start with some simple data aggregation techniques that help us to describe and find patterns in qualitative data by transforming them into more quantitative-like measures.

#### Frequency Counts of Code Categories

Frequency counts and percentages can provide summary statistics of your qualitative data and may assist you in obtaining an overview of your qualitative data as a whole.

- What were the most frequent themes in your data? (It is important to note that the frequency of something may not necessarily relate to its importance, as even the presence of a factor might be qualitatively important.)

- What were the key reasons given for a particular factor of interest to you?

#### Rank Scores

Creating ranked scores is particularly useful if the researcher has structured his or her data so that they can be categorized within and across individual cases (e.g., interviews). You might want to think about the structure of specific cases in your qualitative component so that you might take advantage of quantizing your data later. It might be helpful to ask yourself the following questions:

- Does the collection of your qualitative data allow you to structure your specific cases?

- Have you asked specific questions in your interviews that will allow the categorizing of your data into relevant descriptive categories, for example, by social class or race?

As you analyze your data, you may find that they can be structured in other useful ways as specific categories that you find relevant emerge. You might think about obtaining a consultation with a statistician so that you are clear on what statements you can make about your data in a transformed state. You might also want to build in the possibility of scoring specific categories by asking respondents to provide their own assessments of a given set of issues. An alternative to ranking the data is to ask respondents to rank the data themselves. This would involve asking questions that explore personal salience by asking respondents to order their preferences, perceptions, behaviors, and so forth.

### More Complex Data Transformations: Creating Typologies from Qualitative Data

The following is a more specific empirical example that demonstrates how a qualitative approach to mixed methods utilizes quantitative data transformation techniques to quantize qualitative data. Hesse-Biber (1996) formulated a study concerning the eating habits and body image concerns of white college women. She interviewed a purposive sample of 55 women and had them fill out a self-administered survey in order to explore the following question: Is there a relationship between critical remarks from family and friends and the development of eating-disordered symptoms among women?

Hesse-Biber created an "eating typology" based on the quantitative data that developed from the qualitative data. This quantitative typology led to the creation of quantitative categories that improved the findings' generalizability. The findings show that although some peers and families are supportive of the participants' weight and body image, some are very critical of the young women. The following excerpts were taken from several of the interviews Hesse-Biber conducted (1996, as cited in Hesse-Biber & Leavy, 2006e, p. 328). In this first excerpt, note how Joanna's mother is supportive of her body image:

"My mother, all she wants is that I'm happy. I can weigh 500 pounds as long as I'm happy. Her focus was always on my health, not so much with my appearance. So her comments were more toward always that positive support. Very rarely do I remember her giving like negative comments about how I looked. It was mostly encouraging. My mother would say stuff like 'You have a beautiful face, you have beautiful hands.' She'd focus on individual qualities about me."

On the other side, Joan and Becky received negative responses from their families on their weight and body images:

JOAN: "My brothers and sisters would go around and make pig noises. . . . My dad would say, 'You need to lose weight.' And I'd try and I'd be successful."

BECKY: "My brothers would mention to my mother, and she would say, 'Rob thinks you are getting fat,' and then she'd say, 'Maybe you should stop eating so much.' He [father] commented a lot. Never bad. Always good. He'd say, 'You look good, you lost weight.' He was always commenting on pretty young girls. So I knew it was important to him that I look good too. I wanted him to see that I could be as pretty as all the girls he was commenting on. I wanted him to be proud of me for that and I knew he was."

It is difficult to establish causal relationships in a 55-person sample, and it was increasingly difficult to try to answer a quantitative question using qualitative analysis. Though a lot of qualitative information was gathered about the women's experiences, Hesse-Biber (1996) had trouble establishing a causal relationship between critical attitudes of peers and parents (the cause, or independent variable) and the presence of an eating disorder in the respondent (the effect, or the dependent variable).

By quantizing the qualitative data, the qualitative data (codes) could be transformed into quantitative data (variables). The process of quantizing the data works in the following ways, as illustrated by the procedures followed in Hesse-Biber's (1996) study:

■ *Step 1: Code the text.* In order to help identify key patterns in the series of interviews, Hesse-Biber coded them using HyperRESEARCH, a qualitative data analysis software program (Hesse-Biber et al., 1991). Coding allows you to find patterns by organizing and reducing your data through labeling segments of the text. It develops higher-level codes (*themes*) and uses the process of *memoing* to locate larger meanings related to the research problem. The researchers' main goal in coding is to find larger themes or significant patterns of meaning in the data by grouping, comparing, and contrasting various codes. For example, Joan's comment concerning her family, "My dad would say, 'You need to lose weight,' " was given the qualitative code "parents or peers or siblings critical" (PPSC).

■ *Step 2: Convert codes into variables (qualitative to quantitative).* Relevant qualitative codes were then transformed into quantitative binary variables (variables with only one value: 1 = "present" or 0 = "absent"). In this case, it was noted that 16 of the 55 women reported that a parent, peer, or sibling was critical of their bodies (PPSC). These reports were assigned the value of 1 ("yes"). The other 39 respondents, who did not indicate any form of critical feedback from their parents, siblings, or peers, were assigned a value of 0 ("no"). This same process was also conducted to obtain a binary variable for the presence of an eating disorder (EATDIS; see Hesse-Biber & Carter, 2004, p. 89, for a more detailed account). Table 3.1 displays a matrix of quantized binary variables.

■ *Step 3: Analyze the data.* The CAQDAS program exports these *variables* (qualitative codes transformed into variables) as a matrix in order to obtain a table of values for each of the relevant quantized binary variables. A more detailed statistical analysis of these data is then performed, depending on what the researcher wants to explore.

Hesse-Biber (Hesse-Biber, 1996; Hesse-Biber & Carter, 2004) analyzed the relationship between eating disorders (EATDIS) and the critical remarks of parents, peers, and siblings (PPSC) and constructed Table 3.2. Specifically, this table shows a strong relationship between PPSC and reported eating disorder symptoms such as bulimia and anorexia (EATDIS).

Hesse-Biber (1996) elaborated on this relationship by looking at other quantized variables that might be related to this finding and, seeking further validation of the finding, sought other factors that may have weakened or strengthened the original bivariate relationships found between criticism and eating disorder symptoms. She added a third variable measuring whether or not a parent was overweight and critical of his or her daughter's body. Interestingly enough, she found that whereas criticism from a parent who was not

**TABLE 3.1.** Quantizing Data: Transforming Codes into Variables

| | Interview No. | | | | | | | | | | | | | | | |
|---|---|---|---|---|---|---|---|---|---|---|---|---|---|---|---|---|
| | 1 | 2 | 3 | 4 | 5 | 6 | 7 | 8 | 9 | 10 | 11 | 12 | 13 | 14 | 15 | 16 |
| EATDIS<br>0 = no, 1 = yes | 0 | 0 | 1 | 1 | 0 | 1 | 1 | 0 | 0 | 1 | 1 | 0 | 0 | 0 | 0 | 1 |
| PPSC<br>0 = no, 1 = yes | 0 | 1 | 1 | 1 | 1 | 1 | 0 | 1 | 0 | 0 | 0 | 1 | 0 | 0 | 0 | 1 |

*Note.* Only the first 16 cases of the study are shown as an illustration.

**TABLE 3.2.** Linking Qualitative and Quantitative Data in a Bivariate Table: The Relationship between Having an Eating Disorder and Growing Up with Parents, Peers, or Siblings "Critical" of One's Body and Eating Habits

|         | PPSC | |
|---------|------|------|
| EATDIS  | No   | Yes  |
| Yes     | 12.8 (5)  | 56.3 (9)  |
| No      | 87.2 (34) | 43.8 (7)  |
| Total   | 100% (39) | 100% (16) |

*Note. n = 55.*

overweight was associated with a daughter's eating disorder, criticism from an overweight parent was not, suggesting that the critical words of an overweight parent had less power to produce an eating disorder in daughters than criticism from a parent who was not overweight. Tables 3.3 and 3.4 display this additional information.

By quantizing qualitative data, Hesse-Biber (1996) was able to specifically point to the particular conditions that either strengthen or weaken the relationship between critical responses and eating disorder symptoms. (The variable was whether at least one parent was overweight.) Hesse-Biber and Leavy (2006e) noted finding

> interaction between PPSC and having an overweight parent (or not) in determining the likelihood of an interviewee developing an eating disorder. More specifically, we find that PPSC only really matters in the context of a family where the parents are *not* overweight. In sum, having a critical parent who is at the same time overweight seems to have little impact on a daughter developing an eating disorder, whereas a daughter with parents who are

**TABLE 3.3.** Linking Qualitative and Quantitative Data in a Bivariate Table with Another Quantized Variable: The Relationship between Having an Eating Disorder and Growing Up with Parents, Peers, or Siblings "Critical" of One's Body and Eating Habits for Those Interviewees *Not* Having an Overweight Parent

|         | PPSC | |
|---------|------|------|
| EATDIS  | No   | Yes  |
| Yes     | 7.1 (2)   | 66.7 (8)  |
| No      | 92.9 (26) | 33.3 (4)  |
| Total   | 100% (28) | 100% (12) |

*Note. n = 40.*

**TABLE 3.4.** Linking Qualitative and Quantitative Data in a Bivariate Table with Another Quantized Variable: The Relationship between Having an Eating Disorder and Growing Up with Parents, Peers, or Siblings "Critical" of One's Body and Eating Habits for Those Interviewees Having at Least One Overweight Parent

| | PPSC | |
| --- | --- | --- |
| EATDIS | No | Yes |
| Yes | 27.3 (3) | 25.0 (1) |
| No | 72.7 (8) | 75.0 (3) |
| Total | 100% (11) | 100% (4) |

*Note. n* = 15.

both "thinnish" and *critical* has a strong likelihood of developing bulimia or anorexia. (pp. 329–330)

## APPENDIX 3.2. Qualitizing Quantitative Data

In addition, the mixed methods component of CAQDAS allows the qualitizing of quantitative data. Qualitizing serves to (1) enhance the researcher's understanding of the quantitative data by placing it in a qualitative context, creating a "hybrid" analysis, and (2) provide researchers with a set of variables with which to sort their qualitative data into quantitative categories to enhance the generalizability of their findings. A researcher who qualitizes her or his data may want to enhance her or his understanding of quantitative variables by nesting these variables in a qualitative context.

Hesse-Biber's (1996) study on women's body image and eating disorders contained both qualitative and quantitative data. She conducted intensive interviews with a sample of women 2 years after college and followed up this interview by having her respondents fill out a self-administered questionnaire regarding women's attitudes toward eating, as well as a range of quantitative eating-disorder scales right after the intensive interview component. The interviews and questionnaires were connected for each respondent in her study. She created an "eating typology" based on the quantitative data. The qualitative data from the intensive interviews provided a more detailed "grounding" of the meaning of the eating typology Hesse-Biber created. In addition, the quantitative typology provided her with quantitative categories with which to differentiate her qualitative sample and to enhance the generalizability of her findings regarding women's eating patterns. Hesse-Biber (1996) used insights from the quantitative study to make inferences about the qualitative data. The following are some steps to consider as you begin to qualitize your quantitative data:

■ *Step 1: Collect data.* Here are a series of questions you might ask in the process of qualitizing: How will you collect your quantitative data? Alongside the qualitative data (in the same study) or in different studies? Which will you collect first? Should you collect each type of data over time (longitudinal mixed methods design)? You can collect both quantitative and qualitative data within the same study (Time 1) or sequentially, collecting these data in two separate studies (Time 1 and Time 2). You might even decide to collect one or both types of data at multiple time points. Thus time becomes one of the dimensions in how you collect data.

Hesse-Biber (1996) collected both types of data in the same study. She conducted in-depth interviews with a sample of women 2 years after college regarding issues of body image and eating attitudes (QUAL) and respondents in the study also filled out a structured questionnaire on eating attitudes (QUAN), which she gave them right after the in-depth interview.

You will notice that both of these types of data are capitalized (QUAL and QUAN). Hesse-Biber (1996) considered both types of data to be primary. This was an analysis decision based on her research problem. She did not privilege one type of data over the other. However, this is but one of the many ways you might combine qualitative and quantitative data, and it raises the issue of how to integrate both types of data into your analysis. Questions of integration go to the heart of what it means to qualitize your quantitative data.

■ *Step 2: Determine how you will integrate your quantitative variables into a qualitative study.* There are varieties of ways to do this. Qualitizing involves bringing quantitative variables into interaction with qualitative data (usually in the form of qualitative codes). Some reasons for doing so include *triangulation* and *clarification* of your research concepts. Ask yourself the following: Do you want to use quantitative data to inform your qualitative data or vice versa?

These two approaches make for different ways of qualitizing. The first has to do with using quantitative variables within a qualitative study to inform or provide a more in-depth understanding about the meaning of qualitative codes. Let's go back to Hesse-Biber's (1996) study. She brought in respondents' test scores on the Eating Attitudes Test (EAT) and the Eating Disorders Inventory (EDI) to create a quantitative dichotomous variable called Eating Disorders (ED) that has two categories, "yes" and "no." She wanted to understand the extent to which this quantitative variable corresponded to a similar measure she had derived from her qualitative data on eating disorders, an inductive category titled EATDIS (eating disorders). Where was there agreement (triangulation on this concept) or disagreement? The answer might help her to clarify the meaning of her qualitative code, EATDIS. The purpose was to help inform the meaning of her qualitative codes.

The question of disagreement involves the "meaning" of a quantitative variable in a qualitative context. What does it mean for a respondent to score high on the ED variable? We might use the ED variable to sort respondents by a number of qualitative body image codes in order to get a more in-depth understanding of the context in which individuals talk about their eating issues by ED categories. By contextualizing our quantitative variable, we are able to obtain more clarity of meaning through grounding this variable in a specific social context.

Here you would use quantitative variables to sort through your qualitative codes. Hesse-Biber (1996) used her quantitative variables to make some generalizations about her qualitative findings; for example, she used the ED variable to see what qualitative codes might be related.

## GLOSSARY

**codes:** labels (descriptive and/or analytical) given to segments of data taken from a variety of audiovisual or textual sources.

**communicative validity:** those who might be thought of as experts regarding a particular problem get together to evaluate, debate, and discuss the claims or findings of the research.

**ETHNO:** a software program that performs an event structure analysis, examining the timing of specific events.

**HyperRESEARCH:** a multi-media computer-assisted qualitative data analysis software (CAQDAS) program. A cross-platform product that can be used on Windows and Macintosh systems, it contains a theory-generating component that implements grounded theory and mixed methods analysis (see *www.researchware.com* for more details).

**nonrealist tale:** a form of research writing that is less rigid and more concerned with pushing the boundaries of traditional styles. Pays attention to respondents' voices and acknowledges the inherent power dynamics of researcher–researched relationships.

**parallel mixed methods designs:** consist of the concurrent mixing of qualitative and quantitative methods carried out as separate studies within the same research project.

**pragmatic validity:** examines the extent to which research findings affect those studied as well as the wider context within which the study was conducted.

**priority:** the placement of qualitative and quantitative methods as primary or secondary.

**qualitatively driven approach:** an umbrella term used to characterize a variety of approaches: interpretative, feminist, and postmodern. The common core assumption of this approach is that reality is socially constructed and that subjective meaning is a critical component of knowledge building. This approach does not reject outright some notion of objectivity.

**qualitizing:** the transformation of quantitative data such as variable data into qualitative categories.

**quantizing:** the process by which qualitative codes are grouped into variable-like categories that are used as a heuristic device for analyzing qualitative data quantitatively.

**realist tale:** a form of research writing that follows the traditional writing style; the write-up is prepared for publication and often assumes the role of a "true" reflection of a single social reality, with the researcher's individual voice taking a back seat to the "disembodied voice of authority."

**reliability:** whether or not, if the research project's measures were repeated on the same population, it would create the same results both times.

**sequential mixed methods design:** a design in which quantitative and qualitative components are related sequentially in any given study. First one method is employed, and findings from this method serve as input to the next method. The specific ordering of these components gives rise to two basic types of sequential studies. One type is a sequential explanatory design, whereby the quantitative component of a research project is collected and analyzed first and serves as input to a second qualitative component. A second design is a sequential exploratory design in which the qualitative component is first and the quantitative second.

**theoretical framework:** the researcher's theoretical perspective, which is critical to the building of a mixed methods design and may or may not be explicitly stated in the research.

**validity:** whether or not a method's findings represent the phenomenon they are supposed to measure.

## DISCUSSION QUESTIONS

1. What form of mixed methods design is often used to triangulate qualitative data? In what way is it used?

2. How does one successfully adopt a mixed methodological standpoint? How is this tied to the importance of theory?

3. In deciding on a mixed methods approach, what must be considered in regard to skill level?

4. What are quantizing and qualitizing?

5. What concerns arise from the use of computer software programs in analysis and interpretation?

6. How would you analyze the validity of a qualitatively driven mixed methods research project?

## ■ ■ ■ SUGGESTED WEBSITES ■ ■ ■

### CAQDAS

*www.caqdas.soc.surrey.ac.uk/index.html*

This website provides a wealth of information about using CAQDAS programs in qualitative research.

### Glossary of Mixed Methods Terms/Concepts

*www.fiu.edu/~bridges/glossary.htm*

A list of terms and definitions adopted from Tashakkori and Teddlie's (2003) *Handbook of Mixed Methods in Social and Behavioral Research.*

### Issues in Mixing Qualitative and Quantitative Approaches to Research

*www.researchsupport.com.au/MMIssues.pdf*

This article examines the use of mixed methods and the resulting issues, including demands and paradigmatic problems.

### Qualitatively Driven Mixed Methods

*www.msera.org/Rits_131/Creswell_131.pdf*

This article discusses the important contributions qualitative research makes to mixed methods and draws on leading qualitative and feminist researchers.

## NOTES

1. Although some qualitative approaches embrace a more positivistic stance in that they embrace a unitary view of reality, such as that of "classical" ethnography, Denzin and Lincoln (1998) note several types of variations in qualitative research approaches beyond those used by qualitative researchers who may employ a positivistic approach: (1) constructivist–interpretative, (2) critical (Marxist, emancipatory), and (3) feminist (p. 33). A *constructivist or interpretative paradigm* sees reality as subjective, consisting of stories or meanings produced or constructed by individuals within their "natural" settings. A *critical paradigm* deals with how power, control, and ideology dominate our understanding of reality. A *postmodernist paradigm* examines how social life is produced and privileged by those in power. The goal of knowledge building is to "emancipate" and to expose social injustice. For postmodernists, reality is representational rather than real or "the truth." However, not all critical theorists take such a relativistic stance on truth. *Feminist perspectives* stress the importance of understanding women's lived experiences. Feminist researchers concern themselves with issues not only of gender but also of race, class, ethnicity, sexual orientation, and so forth. Feminist researchers seek subjugated knowledge by exposing the hidden voices of women. These varying theoretical perspectives, subsets of a general qualitative approach, often remain marginalized and stereotyped, with little discussion of the myriad rich research that is going on within and between these perspectives as they relate to the mixed methods research represented in more mainstream journals and books on the topic.

2. For a list of major commercial software for qualitative data analysis, refer to the CAQDAS website listed at the end of this chapter.

3. Fuzzy-set theory (see Ragin, 2000) questions long-held ideas of group membership. Ragin (2000) described a "fuzzy set" as troubling positivistic categorization. He provided the example of the issues involved in categorizing quantitative data, applying a socially constructed viewpoint to the process of categorization. The idea of creating binary categorizations of any category becomes limiting and fails to capture any given individual perceptions. Statistically turning a binary category into a continuous one

is problematic, as it remains ungrounded in a social context. Ragin (2000) noted: "The fuzzy set is much more than a 'continuous' variable because it is much more heavily infused with theoretical and substantive knowledge . . . a fuzzy set is more empirically grounded and more precise" (p. 6).

4. This section is adapted from Hesse-Biber and Leavy (2006f). Copyright 2006 by Sage Publications, Inc. Adapted by permission.

5. Appendix 3.1 is adapted in part from Hesse-Biber and Leavy (2006a). Copyright 2006 by Sage Publications, Inc. Adapted by permission.

# CHAPTER 4

# Interpretative Approaches to Mixed Methods Research

An interpretative approach to research aims to understand how individuals make meaning of their social world. The social world is not something independent of individual perceptions but is created through social interactions of individuals with the world around them. This approach is committed to multiple views of social reality. An interpretative approach can be considered conterminous with a qualitative approach in general. The linkage between the two is often cited as distinguishing the interpretative from a quantitative approach to research, which one often associates with the use of statistical analysis and large-scale datasets. Yet what distinguishes an interpretative approach is not what methods it uses—qualitative, textual data, for example, or quantitative analysis; rather, the distinction lies in considering the ontological and epistemological standpoint the researcher brings to bear in his or her social inquiry.

Figure 4.1 highlights the range of philosophical standpoints with regard to ontology and epistemology, depicted along a continuum. Although many qualitative approaches favor the subjective standpoint and although those who practice a "positivistic" approach tend more toward the objective end of this continuum, there are many researchers whose basic philosophical standpoints lie between the two.

An interpretative approach harks back to our discussion of the importance of considering the ontological and epistemological standpoint of the researcher. The interpretative approach does not accept the

Subjective ←――――――――――→ Objective

| | Subjective | Objective |
|---|---|---|
| **Ontology:** What is the nature of the reality? | Social reality is multiple. | There is a concrete social world "out there." |
| **Epistemology:** What can we know and who can know? | Goal is to understand multiple subjectivities. Individuals are the "experts." Through intersubjectivity we understand human behaviors. There is no definitive subject–object split in knowledge building. | Goal is to ascertain the "truth" in order to predict and even uncover "laws" of human behavior through objective social inquiry. Scientists are the experts. |

**FIGURE 4.1.** Philosophical standpoints in the research.

idea of an "objective reality" that a positivistic approach takes as given. For the interpretative researcher, the social reality is created through the social interactions of individuals with the world around them. A mixed methods project from an interpretative perspective often uses quantitative research as an auxiliary to a primary qualitative methodology as a means of both understanding the broader objective context and contextualizing people's experiences.

This chapter presents several examples of interpretative approaches that utilize a variety of mixed methods designs. We present the range of reasons that researchers employ an interpretative approach to mixed methods designs and the process by which they do so. Lastly, we touch on some of the problems and perils they confront in the process.

## The Practice of an Interpretative Approach to Mixed Methods Research: Case Studies

The following case studies of mixed methods from an interpretative approach often employ a *sequential mixed methods design,* that is, a research design that begins with either a quantitative study followed by a qualitative study or a qualitative study followed by a quantitative study.

An *explanatory sequential design* (see Figure 4.2) is one in which the collection and analysis of quantitative data is followed by the collection and analysis of qualitative data. Creswell et al. (2003) note that this design gives priority to the quantitative aspects of the study. However, from the perspective of an interpretive approach, researchers view the quantitative component as in the service of the qualitative component, which is considered primary.[1] An *exploratory sequential design* (see Chapter 3, Figure 3.2), on the other hand, begins with a qualitative data collection and analysis followed by a quantitative study. This design gives priority to the qualitative aspects of the research project (Creswell et al., 2003).

We observe sequential designs, both exploratory and explanatory, that give priority to the interpretive approach. Methods do not define

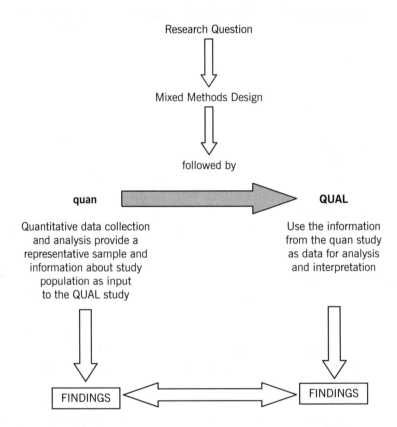

**FIGURE 4.2.** quan → QUAL explanatory sequential study. The double arrow signifies the following: (1) researchers can go back from the QUAL to the quan findings to see to what extent the QUAL findings compare with the wider quan population, increasing "generalizability and validity"; and (2) in those cases in which the same or similar questions are linked between the studies, the researcher may assess validity through *triangulation* of results. One could also examine contradictions between quan and QUAL data in order to generate new research questions or insight.

what takes priority; an understanding of research design gives deter-mination of priority to the research question. The role that methods collection and analysis take on in a sequential design must come from the overall research problem. Seen in this light, interpretative research-ers may often use an explanatory sequential design to generate theory. Therefore, a researcher might employ a quantitative study first to provide a more representative sample as input into her or his primary qualitative study in order to produce a more valid study and a more robust way of generating theory. Researchers can use an exploratory sequential study to test theory by using the theoretical insights gained in the qualitative study in a larger quantitative study. There are myriad sequential designs and motivations that may come about, making the process of mixing methods more an iterative than a static process. Given this iterative quality of mixing methods from an interpretative approach, employing a sequential design hinges on the research question, as well as the ways in which data collection and analysis of both sets of data interact to lead to the asking of additional questions, and so on.

In this chapter I present several case studies of interpretative approaches to mixed methods research. In the analysis of each study, we address several sensitizing questions:

- How can a mixed methods design further the goals of an inter-pretative approach to understanding social reality?

- Why and how do interpretative researchers employ mixed meth-ods across the research process at (1) the data gathering stage, (2) the data analysis stage, and (3) the qualitative stage?

### Case Study 1: Studying the Experience of Being a Teenager

Julia Brannen and her colleagues (Brannen, Dodd, Oakley, & Storey, 1994) conducted a mixed methods study on the health and family life of teenagers. They sought to answer some critical research questions:

- What is it like to be a teenager today?

- How do parents and teenagers experience their roles and respon-sibilities?

- How does the promotion of health and responsibility figure in the perspectives and priorities of young people and their par-ents?

- Under what circumstances do young people assume responsibility for their health?

- How do parents try to minimize teen risk taking, and are they successful?

Their study was conducted in two phases. The first phase consisted of distributing a self-administered survey to 843 fifteen- and sixteen-year-olds in schools in a multiethnic West London borough. It is at this critical age, the authors noted, that teens are "making important decisions concerning their future education, training and employment" (1994, p. 8). The goal of the quantitative survey was to provide an overview of the general health of this population and, in turn, compare these findings with those from a national population, as the researchers modeled the survey after a national health questionnaire administered throughout the United Kingdom (p. 8).

The second phase consisted of in-depth interviews taken from a subsample of teens who were randomly chosen from the survey respondents. The authors interviewed teens and their parents from a total of 64 households (142 interviews total), which included the respondent and, where possible, both parents. By using the household as their unit of analysis, as well as looking at individual teens' experiences, the researchers had a micro context within which they could assess how a teenager's experience of health and illness plays out in the social context of his or her own household (including values, attitudes, and actions of their parents).

The researchers made clear that their use of mixed methods was in the service of addressing different issues. The survey provided a wider context for understanding teens' health behaviors and their demographic backgrounds. More important, the survey also provided researchers with a *sampling frame* of the larger population that enabled them to select a random sample for their study. This strategy permitted Brannen and colleagues (1994) to generalize the findings to the larger population and to represent its full ethnic diversity. They noted that "the interviewed group reflects the ethnic composition of the questionnaire sample reasonably well" and that "the wide variation in household composition almost exactly reflects the distribution in the questionnaire survey" (Brannen et al., 1994, p. 15).

The researchers selected several survey questions to bring into their qualitative study so that they might continually link findings from the interviews to the more general survey population in order to make more specific statements about how the findings from their in-depth study might be generalized to the wider population, thereby strengthening the validity of their findings. They accomplished this linking by weaving quantitative findings into their analysis of the qualitative data results. They juxtaposed the in-depth findings with their survey results, especially in those instances in which the qualitative and quantitative data collected similar information. For example, they asked teens in both studies about taking responsibility for their health. In the survey questionnaire, teens were more likely to report that their parents took responsibility for their health (e.g., monitoring "diet and personal cleanliness"), but in the in-depth interview teens were more likely to say that they themselves took responsibility for their own health (1994, p. 208). In another instance, teens reported a higher degree of drug use in the survey than they did in the in-depth interviews (1994, p. 121).

This is noteworthy because the authors stated that the time lag between the survey and the in-depth interview was between 6 and 15 months, with the quantitative study being conducted first (p. 120). During this time period, changes could have occurred in teens' risk-taking behaviors; additionally, the questionnaire, with its relative anonymity, could have provided a safer venue for teens to talk about their risk-taking behaviors. The time difference between the studies' two components complicates the results because the respondents provided different information according to their conditions at each time (p. 77).

Such discrepancies in the findings were not dismissed but gave rise to important issues regarding reliability of in-depth findings and the best way to collect different types of data. The authors note that "these differences between questionnaire and interview data are . . . important if the aim is to obtain the most reliable estimates possible of young people's health-related behaviours" (Brannen et al., 1994, p. 121).

This juxtaposition of findings from each type of dataset also allowed the researchers to enhance the validity of their findings. Although the questions were not exactly the same, the authors were able to speculate about the generalizability of their findings by comparing them with more general survey findings on a similar issue. For example, they compared a survey question about young people's relationships with their parents with the corresponding interview questions. In addition, the findings also served to elaborate the survey results by providing a more complex understanding of teens' family relationships by examining the experiences of all three family members—teens, mothers, and fathers; and, in doing so, they uncovered the intensity and importance of mothers (especially with regard to the mother–daughter dyad) and the more peripheral role of fathers in their children's health-related care.

The design of Brannen et al.'s study can be labeled "mixed methods sequential explanatory." We can see in Figure 4.3 that the quantitative study enables the researchers to select cases for their qualitative study such that the mixed methods design is sequential—quan followed by QUAL—where the qualitative component is primary (although it comes second) and the quantitative study provides input (a sample of selected cases) for the interviews. However, at the data analysis stage, the findings from both QUAL and quan are in conversation with each other in a variety of ways.

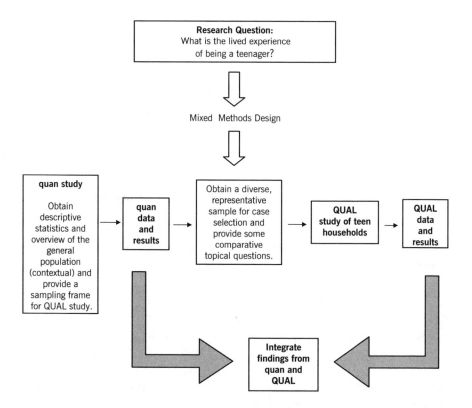

**FIGURE 4.3.** Study of health and family life of teenagers: Mixed methods explanatory sequential study.

### Case Study 2: Understanding the Recreational Constraints on Families with Disabled Children

Jennifer Mactavish's (Mactavish & Schleien, 2004) study of family recreation provides another example of how researchers utilize quantitative methods in the service of qualitative questions. Using a qualitative paradigm—what Mactavish terms a "naturalistic/constructivist" model (Guba & Lincoln, 1994)—the authors seek to understand how families with developmentally disabled children perceive "the nature and benefits of, and constraints to, family recreation" (Mactavish & Schleien, 2004, p. 123).

Similar to the study by Brannen et al. (1994), discussed in the preceding section, the first phase of Mactavish and Schleien's (2004) research project was quantitative: They administered a survey questionnaire to a sample of parents with disabled children. This questionnaire contained open- and closed-ended questions derived from previous research literature on the general topic of recreation. The purpose of this initial survey was to provide the researchers with a context within which to understand the data they gathered in the second phase of the project. In addition, the survey data also provided them with some answers to a variety of topical questions addressed in the study. They noted, "the questionnaire data provided initial insights about a breadth of family recreation topics and, in turn, became the foundation for the interviews" (p. 126). Note that this sequence of using quantitative survey questions as an aid to the development of a qualitative study is a reversal of the usual emphasis in mixed methods research.

A second goal, similar to the previous case study on adolescent health, was to recruit a sample of families with disabled children for the research project. This also allowed the researchers subsequently to link their study to the quantitative component of their research. They write:

> [the] questionnaire included an invitation to participate in a series of follow-up interviews. Forty-four families expressed an interest in being interviewed, and from this pool, 16 were ultimately selected using a sequential–purposive sampling technique. . . . That is, the first eight families were selected using a criterion approach, which sought to ensure that those interviewed reflected the overall sociodemographic diversity of the sample. As analyses began to produce patterns related to the research questions of interest, eight additional families were selected based on consistencies between their questionnaire responses and emerging interpretations of the inter-

view data (i.e., a theory-based purposive technique). (Mactavish & Schleien, 2004, p. 126)[2]

What Mactavish and Schleien noted, then, is that they used the quantitative component to increase the generalizability of their study in a few ways. First, it provided them with a sample that reflected the wider population of families with developmentally disabled children. Second, it allowed them to explore various theoretical ideas they had regarding disability by using interviews to explore in greater depth theoretically relevant patterns found in the quantitative data, such as "who participates [in recreation] and where this takes place" and what "specific activities" the families engage in (pp. 129–130). In this sense, the authors were able to capitalize on the quantitative findings but remain open and flexible in the study. They noted that "the interviews were used to intensively explore issues arising from the questionnaires while being flexible enough to accommodate emerging issues and questions" (p. 127).

In terms of the analysis of their data, Mactavish and Schleien (2004) appear to favor the goal of triangulation (see Figure 4.4), namely looking at how their qualitative study agreed with or confirmed their quantitative findings. What appears to be a lesser priority in this project is looking at how the findings diverged from or contradicted one another and how these tensions in the results could help the researchers to pose new problems and issues that need to be addressed in future research studies.

The next two briefly reported case studies are included to explain how the use of the quantitative component of a mixed methods design can assist an interpretative approach in terms of enabling the researcher to gather a purposive sample for a qualitative study. The quantitative study provides a way for researchers to sample specific informants who are likely to exemplify patterns that the researcher will pursue in an in-depth qualitative study.

### Case Study 3: Studying Violence against Women

Frost (1999), a British researcher, wanted to understand perceptions of domestic violence from the point of view of health personnel—in particular, those who made home health visits to female clients' homes. A questionnaire was sent to two National Health Service (NHS) trusts, one in London and another in southeast England, which provided care

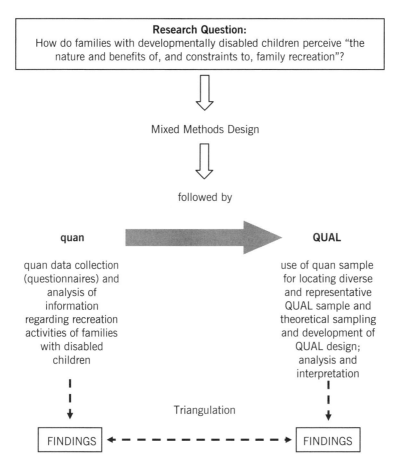

**FIGURE 4.4.** The family recreation and developmental disability study: Sequential design (with goals of generalizability and triangulation).

to 134 recipients. The questionnaire provided both data on the extent of domestic violence (by ascertaining the number of abused women identified by health practitioners in their practice) and a means to recruit a small sample of health practitioners for a follow-up in-depth study. From the larger quantitative study, Frost was able to select a *purposive sample* of visiting health personnel who were involved with women who had experienced violence and who had children of preschool age.

A second example of this type of mixed methods design is provided by Gerbert, Abercrombie, Caspers, Love, and Bronstone (1999), who wanted to understand battered women's perceptions of the barriers to seeking and finding medical assistance. Gerbert and colleagues employed qualitative and quantitative methods in their study. Quantitative methods were used to obtain a purposive sample of battered women, as well as to provide some information on prevalence rates of abuse. The quantitative study consisted of a sample of 334 women who had been victims of physical violence within the past year, and data were gathered through random-digit dialing. At this time, those women sampled were also administered a Conflict Tactics Scale (CTS) to ascertain their levels of abuse. The quantitative findings were analyzed, and those individuals who met the CTS criteria for abuse were then selected for a second study (the qualitative component of the mixed methods design), in which women were interviewed using an open-ended questionnaire regarding their intimate relationships, chronology of abuse, and experience in obtaining health care after an abuse incident.

The use of a quantitative component first in this mixed methods design is especially important in uncovering a "hard to find" target population. Domestic abuse is a hidden problem, and beginning with a large quantitative study provides the researchers with more possibilities of finding women who have faced abuse. In addition, the anonymity of a larger survey may, in fact, increase the response rate. Trying to locate a sample like this by using more qualitative techniques, such as snowball referral sampling, may be inappropriate given the private nature of this social problem.

### Case Study 4: Understanding Influences on Nutritional Awareness among Low-Income Clients

In this mixed methods project, Brian Grim and his colleagues (Grim, Harmon, & Gromis, 2006) were interested in understanding how newsletters on nutrition distributed at food pantries for low-income men and women affected the nutritional awareness of their clients. They wrote:

> Projects working with food pantries usually provide nutrition education when food is distributed to clients. Of the different ways that such education can be provided, nutrition newsletters are frequently used since they provide a cost-effective way to provide information to all clients. Because of the ubiquitous use of newsletters to accomplish this education aim, the relevance of their content, the appeal of their design, and the circumstances of their distribution are important issues to better understand. (Grim et al., 2006, p. 519, footnote 3)

Grim et al.'s (2006) mixed methods research design consisted of embedding a quantitative method within an ongoing qualitative study (Figure 4.5). The study was primarily qualitative but utilized a quantitative method to enhance the understanding of respondents' experiences. More specifically, Grim and his colleagues incorporated a quantitative method into a focus-group format. One of the important issues in conducting a focus group is knowing when you have exhausted a topic, such that further elaboration on a given topic no longer produces new information. To help with the issue of *topic saturation*, the researchers used an experiment-like component that they embedded in their ongoing focus-group interviews and that allowed them to determine when and how a topic became saturated within a focus group (p. 517). In this specific focus-group interview, they were interested in which informational format was most effective in aiding participants' understanding of safety information regarding how to handle meat products and whether, in fact, a newsletter was the best way to convey this information.

Instead of focusing on only the conversational element within the focus group as a means of finding out the possible ways of thinking about how information was best conveyed about this particular topic, Grim et al. (2006) decided to have focus-group participants take time out of their ongoing conversation to read three articles that discussed how to thaw meat, asking respondents to read each of the articles without discussion. Each participant was then asked individually to determine which of these three articles gave the "most practical advice on thawing a large piece of meat" (p. 522). They scored the respondents' choices out loud, and the moderator then asked the participants to dis-

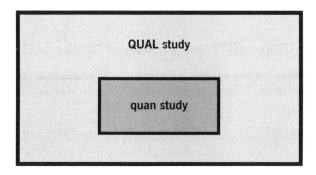

**FIGURE 4.5.** A quantitative study embedded within a qualitative study: Study of nutritional awareness among low-income clients.

cuss and decide among themselves what was the most practical advice they had gotten from reading the articles. After discussing their opinions, participants were asked to vote again on what article was most practical and why. This process continued until the group secured consensus on this issue.

In doing this embedded quantitative intervention in a primarily qualitative study, these researchers were able to get at new information by accessing it through the use of another method. Both the qualitative and quantitative components of this project acted in the service of a qualitative approach. What is novel about this mixed methods design is that respondents can articulate meaning using both words and numbers. There is a close interrelationship between the results of each type of inquiry; they support the goals of getting at respondents' meanings and understanding a specific phenomenon.

Grim et al. (2006) call this type of analysis "quanti–qualitative" methodology (p. 531). The authors seek to enhance the overall understanding of their problem through the use of both qualitative and quantitative analyses and interpretation of their focus-group data.

### Case Study 5: Comparing the Lived Occupational Experiences of Baby-Boomer and Generation X Physicians

The following case study began as an exploratory research project and utilized a mixed methods qualitative approach to draw out information regarding the shifts in the medical field between baby-boomer and Generation X physicians. Jovic, Wallace, and Lemaire's (2006) study started out with several questions on generation and gender shifts in medicine, namely:

1. How do baby-boomer and Generation X physicians perceive the generational shift in work attitudes and behaviors?

2. Do baby-boomer and Generation X physicians differ significantly in their work hours and work attitudes regarding patient care and life balance?

3. Do female and male Generation X physicians differ significantly in their work hours and work attitudes regarding patient care and life balance? (p. 1)

The authors' research goal was exploratory, and they conducted a mixed methods exploratory sequential design. They began by conducting 54 in-depth interviews with a quota sample "based on gender, division, rank, site/hospital affiliation, scholarly activity and family status" of baby-boomer doctors (those born between 1946 and 1964) and Generation X doctors (those born between 1965 and 1980; p. 3). They followed up with a mail survey to all physicians and residents in the "university and health region based Department of Medicine in a large, metropolitan city in Western Canada" (p. 3). The in-depth interviews were used to answer the first question, and the survey interviews were designed to answer the second and third questions.

The results of the qualitative study revealed that baby-boomer doctors perceived the younger generation to work fewer hours, thereby being able to have more balanced work and family lives, a practice that they felt meant that the younger generation was less committed to the medical field than their own generation. On the other hand, Generation X physicians felt that they were strongly committed to medicine and did not perceive working more hours as a sign of commitment to medicine. They reported striving for a more balanced work–family commitment (Jovic et al., 2006).

The analysis of results from the quantitative study, which measured the actual number of reported hours worked and perceived balance between work and family, revealed that, despite their perceptions to the contrary, both generations reported "similar attitudes and experiences with respect to patient care and work–life balance . . . and . . . both generations average 61 work hours a week" (p. 7). The survey data also revealed that Generation X physicians had a difficult time in balancing their work and family commitments, very similar to the information reported by baby boomers, with the exception that boomers "seem to view the relationship between the work and family domains as zero-sum, or independent, where greater commitment to one means less commitment to the other" (p. 7). In addition, Jovic et al. (2006) compared results by gender for Generation X physicians; enough women and men were in medicine at that time to compare the genders.[3] The authors found little difference in the work attitudes and experiences, as well as the work hours and commitment to patient care, between men and women of Generation X. They did find, however, that women doctors experienced a greater lack of balance in their work and family commitments.

The authors brought together the findings from their qualitative and quantitative data in their overall interpretation of research results and noted that, despite the perceptions of difference between the generations of doctors, there was a similar degree of professional commitment: "These similarities may reflect the extensive professional social-ization that physicians receive throughout their medical training that promotes the internalization of the same core work values and behav-iors associated with practicing medicine, regardless of which genera-tion they belong to" (Jovic et al., 2006, p. 7).

The use of a mixed methods design expands our understanding of the contradictory perceptions of the work–family experiences of Gener-ation X physicians through their own eyes and through the eyes of the baby-boomer generation. These generational perceptions are quite dif-ferent. The quantitative component of the mixed methods design helps to sort out the validity of these generational perceptions and provides the researcher with a way of placing these different findings in a wider sociohistorical context. But more than this, the mixed methods results also reveal an ideological generational fissure within the medical pro-fession itself regarding perceptions of occupational expectations of the younger generation of doctors. This gap in understanding may have social policy consequences in that it may place serious barriers in the way of solving the current work–family crisis in medicine described by Generation X doctors, especially among women. The lack of under-standing of the plight of Generation X doctors by baby-boomer doctors may stall the much-needed work–family changes in the medical profes-sion. Many baby-boomer doctors who now occupy positions of power within the medical establishment may not be willing to advocate for more just work–family policies for the younger generation of doctors, whom they feel already have "more balanced" work and family lives. (For a diagram of this type of exploratory sequential mixed methods design, please refer back to Chapter 3, Figure 3.3.)

### Case Study 6: Understanding Perpetrators of Child Sexual Abuse

Gilgun (1992) was interested in studying those factors "which distin-guish adults who are perpetrators of child sexual abuse from persons of similar background who have not acted out sexually with children" (p. 115). Because experiencing childhood sexual abuse is a strong risk factor for becoming an adult perpetrator of sexual abuse, Gilgun com-pared perpetrators with a history of childhood sexual abuse with non-perpetrators with similar histories in order to explore what factors medi-ated the long-term effects of childhood sexual abuse on the likelihood of adult sexual misconduct with children. She conducted a sequential mixed methods study. The qualitative research component of the study came first, allowing the generation of theories and hypotheses. In the following quantitative component, she then tested the theory's general-izability to the population.

The goal of the qualitative component of Gilgun's (1992) research design was to develop an in-depth understanding of behaviors and background characteristics of perpetrators with the goal of generating specific hypotheses about which characteristics distinguished perpetra-tors from nonperpetrators that she could then test on a wider popula-tion. The qualitative component of this study consisted of life history interviews with 41 adults who were abused as children. The author chose a "theoretical sampling" procedure whereby her sample was built "from the ground up," evolving over time by allowing the findings from a prior case analysis to determine what new type of study was needed in order to develop a more complete picture of her research problem. All respondents were volunteers she recruited from several sites, including a maximum-security prison, a medium-security prison, a sexual addic-tion group at a community-based treatment center, and members of a "sex addicts" help group. She cast a wide net to obtain a range of sex offenders in order to build a rich database that would allow her to frame specific hypotheses about the factors associated with sex abuse perpetration.

Gilgun (1992) employed a *grounded theory* method in analyzing her case data that utilized a *constant comparative* method that is built on both induction (generating theory/hypotheses) and deduction (testing the-ory; Glaser & Strauss, 1967). That is, she generated her research ques-tions and hypotheses from her data (induction), testing them against new interview data, as well as relevant research literature (deduction), and modifying her theory/hypotheses in response to new information as her analysis progressed.

Gilgun's (1992) findings revealed several "protective" factors in high-risk individuals that make them resilient and less likely to become violent. She found that having confidants, such as a supportive parent, peer, neighbor, or therapist, for example, plays an important role in mediating the long- and short-term effects of childhood sexual abuse and diminishing the likelihood of becoming a perpetrator as an adult. She also found that women were more likely to have confidants, a find-ing that suggested that this may be one reason that they are less likely to perpetrate as adults. Rather than focusing on traditional "risk models" of violent behavior (i.e., looking at those factors that predict a given individual's risk of becoming a sexual perpetrator), this study focuses on those factors leading to resiliency—that is, those factors (resources) that serve to protect individuals from becoming sexual offenders. In this study, resiliency was indicated by the status of being a nonperpetrating adult despite having a history of sexual abuse as a child. Based on the findings from her study, Gilgun generated several hypotheses, as follows:

- Having confidants is a protective mechanism against becoming a perpetrator of sexual abuse.

- Men who become perpetrators of child sexual abuse use sex to feel better, and, over the life course, they do not have confidants.

- Women are more likely to have confidants and are less likely to use sex to feel better; therefore, they are less at risk than men to become perpetrators of child sexual abuse (p. 122).

In the second phase of her research project, Gilgun and her colleagues Klein and Pranis (2000) used a quantitative approach to test out the generalizability of the "resource theory" model that was discovered in the qualitative component of the mixed methods study. In this regard, two key issues framed the second component of the research project: (1) locating a representative sample of the wider population of sexual offenders and (2) testing out hypotheses regarding the importance of resources in understanding violent sexual behaviors.

The offender sample consisted of 1,311 sexual offenders drawn from the prison population of Minnesota, and the gender, racial, and ethnic composition of this sample represented the overall general prison population. A comparison group of nonoffenders consisted of a random sample of adult males and females ($n = 306$), as well as a sample of adolescent males and females ($n = 1,225$) who were residents of Minnesota (where the primary investigator resided). The adult sample was selected from the University of Minnesota's Annual State Survey, which included "several items representing risks and resources from our questionnaire" (p. 636). An adolescent sample was selected from a stratified random sample of public school students who took part in a National Adolescent Health Survey conducted by the University of Minnesota.

Gilgun et al. (2000) selected several items from the qualitative study to place on the "offender survey" in order to make some specific comparisons. These questions concerned the respondents' early childhood, family structure, relationships at home and with peers, and issues of substance, sexual, and physical abuse.

The quantitative research revealed that those "resource factors" that create resiliency (identified from Gilgun's 1992 study), when added to "risk only" models, were better able to predict offender versus nonoffender groups, as well as to decrease misclassification, such as "offenders classified as nonoffenders (false negatives) and nonoffenders classified as offenders (false positives)" (p. 645). This research is also important because it provides information that can be used to model intervention and prevention of violent behaviors. In this sense the mixed methods design is transformative in that it opens the possibility for social change and new policy initiatives. Gilgun and colleagues (2000) noted:

> Research on risk and resilience has wide-ranging implications for violence prevention and the treatment of perpetrators. Policy makers, program planners, and practitioners are challenged to give increased attention to the resources available to their target populations and to provide them when they are lacking. For example, good experiences in school can offset risks in families and communities. . . . The effectiveness of interventions will greatly increase when professionals turn our attention to resources, as well as risks, and build on positive qualities in individuals, families, institutions, and communities. (p. 647)

Utilizing a mixed methods design allowed Gilgun and colleagues (2000) to generate a more robust theoretical framework for understanding how people may become sexual offenders and provided an opportunity to create interventions to prevent sexual abuse. The qualitative component, consisting of in-depth interviews with both sexual offenders and nonoffenders with histories of childhood sexual abuse, provided the researchers with an opportunity to generate a more robust model of offender behavior by uncovering the significance of resources in preventing offender behaviors. Resources were left out of traditional models of offender behaviors that primarily relied on risk-only models. By listening to offender narratives, the researchers discerned the importance of "resource factors" in individual, family, and community resources that serve to promote resilience. The quantitative component of their project allowed the researchers to test out their theoretical model on a wider population. The results of the quantitative data served to validate their theoretical model by showing that it significantly distinguished between the offender and nonoffender groups better than the risk-only models. Their research project also serves an important transformative goal in that it provides social change agents with the "hard evidence" they need for the prevention of violent behaviors and with specific interventions for those youths already at risk, including working with their families and their local communities.

# Why an Interpretative Approach to Research Uses a Mixed Methods Design

These case studies reveal a range of reasons that researchers who employ an interpretative approach use mixed methods designs. The following is a summary of these reasons, garnered inductively from examining interpretative approaches to mixed methods case studies. I also want to point out that some of these reasons, as we see in the following chapters, are not unique to interpretative mixed methods projects, as these reasons can also overlap to some extent with feminist and postmodern mixed methods rationales for employing a mixed methods design.

### Selecting a Sample

■ *Using a quantitative study to locate a "hard to find" qualitative sample.* The researcher employs a quantitative method in order to reach many people and to target a specific population of interest that may be hard to locate.

■ *Employing a quantitative study in order to increase the generalizability of a qualitative study.* In this regard, starting out with a quantitative study first allows the qualitative researcher to draw a more representative qualitative sample. For example, taking a quantitative demographic survey of a random sample of the researcher's target population enables the researcher to select a subsample from this population that is representative of the target population. This selected qualitative subsample may be directly linked to the quantitative sample or indirectly linked (i.e., the researcher collects a separate sample based on the population characteristics of interest as evidence that the sample is representative because the sample mimics the characteristics of the wider target population).

### Increasing the Validity and Reliability of Qualitative Findings

■ *Drawing a qualitative sample directly or even indirectly from a quantitative sample has the added benefit of increasing the validity and reliability of qualitative findings.* This is especially the case when similar questions are asked in both studies. By linking the methods at the data gathering stage to the qualitative results, the researcher can assess the validity and reliability of the findings. For example, those qualitative researchers who ask similar questions in both the quantitative and qualitative studies are provided with an opportunity to grapple with issues of reliability and validity of research findings by ascertaining (1) the extent to which research findings from similar questions yield similar responses (reliability) and (2) the extent to which their responses appear to get at the same underlying issues such that there is general agreement in their responses (validity through triangulation). The linking of methods also provides an opportunity for the researcher to explore any contradictions in the quantitative study by using a qualitative study to explore these contradictions or to follow up on any unusual results (i.e., the presence of "outliers" in the quantitative study).

■ *Following up with a quantitative study is done in order to test the validity of qualitative findings for a wider population.* The researcher conducts a qualitative study first, followed by a quantitative study that will "test out" the theoretical ideas generated from the qualitative study. In this case, the researcher is interested in ascertaining whether his or her theoretical ideas and findings are generalizable to a larger population.

### Serendipitous Use of Quantitative Findings: The Case of Outliers

■ *A quantitative study may reveal the presence of a subpopulation of "outliers" in the initial target population.* This finding provides an opportunity to expand knowledge regarding the overall research problem and/or generates new problems and questions that require further exploration in a follow-up qualitative research project.

### Serendipitous Use of Quantitative Findings: The Case of Disparate Findings

■ *An originally parallel mixed methods design is expanded to include a follow-up qualitative study that explores disparate findings between the qualitative and quantitative findings.* This procedure may serve to generate new questions that can be explored qualitatively, thereby permitting a more complex understanding of a research problem.

### Using a Quantitative Study to Proactively Enhance the Understanding of the Research Problem and Research Findings

■ *The qualitative researcher deliberately uses a quantitative component as a way to generate new qualitative research questions.* Mixed methods can assist researchers in acquiring specific topical issues and concerns they wish to explore. Here, the quantitative component serves to initiate or spark new hypotheses or research questions that researchers can pursue in depth. In addition, researchers can draw on quantitative findings to explore in more detail issues and discrepancies they may find of interest.

## Challenges to Implementing a Mixed Methods Design and the Need for Researcher Reflexivity

We hope that these case studies that include some of the essential aspects of implementing specific designs have given you a better understanding of the qualitative approach that mixed methods practices can take. However, mixed methods research poses a variety of challenges that also need to be taken into consideration from the outset of a project. For example, as we have seen in several of these case studies, sometimes there is a considerable time lag between the first component of a mixed methods design and the second. This is most pronounced in Gilgun et al.'s research (Gilgun, 1992; Gilgun et al., 2000), in which the studies are linked to each other, but this link spans many years. In fact, this is not an uncommon occurrence in this type of mixed methods design (Bryman, 2007a, p. 14). The time lag is exacerbated when research teams need to regroup and retool as they move from one skills-based method to another. In addition, the resources needed to complete both components may make it difficult to move quickly from one component of a project to another. The researcher may not even be able to integrate her or his findings if the two phases of a project represent a wide time gap. In other circumstances, the time lag might "bring pressures to publish as soon as possible, even though not all the findings have been generated" (Bryman, 2007a, p. 15). As Bryman noted:

> In research teams where there are quantitative and qualitative specialists, where one phase is lagging behind the other, pressure may build up to start publishing the findings that are more advanced.

Typically, this entailed a survey component being much faster to conduct and analyze than a qualitative one. (2007a, p. 14)

Pursuing a qualitative approach to mixed methods design also requires the addition of new research skills and resources, and here it behooves the researcher to question the extent to which she or he may need to retool her or his research skills or to approach the project with a team of differently skilled researchers. The team route to mixed methods does not come without its own set of issues in terms of coordinating how the findings are integrated, if at all (Bryman, 2007a). We take up more of these challenges to mixed methods approaches in the concluding chapter.

Qualitative approaches to mixed methods research privilege the lived experiences of the individuals studied, with the goal of understanding from their perspective. Although we have pointed out the important contributions a quantitative component can bring to a qualitative project, the researcher must be clear on the reasons for the inclusion of a quantitative component, especially because of the special challenges that this type of design poses. More is not necessarily better. There are a variety of reasons for mixing methods, which we discussed, and sometimes these reasons overlap. The practice of mixed methods in social science should be informed by an awareness of the goal of using a combined approach. It may be the case that adding on a quantitative method to a qualitative project does not improve one's theoretical understanding of a given issue. The researcher must be willing to be reflective and ask whether adding a new method will truly serve to enhance qualitative understanding or not.

We leave you with some words of wisdom from Janice Morse, who, in an interview with Cesar Cisneros-Puebla, warns against privileging technique over the larger goal of advancing theory and understanding of social problems in our research simply in order to please funders' current interest in mixed methods research:

> I think the pressure to do mixed methods, in order to get funding overwhelms or overrides the goals of inquiry. . . . I do not think we all have to give into these pressures. I feel I use multi-methods if it is required in the design, not simply to please funding agencies. (quoted in Cisneros-Puebla, 2004, pp. 14–15)

Her words remind us that although mixed methods hold out much promise, they must be used with intentionality and a solid understanding of how their use may advance our goal of meaningful social inquiry.

In the next chapter, we examine the distinctive manner in which feminist qualitative researchers conceptualize and practice mixed methods research in order to address questions about women's lives.

## GLOSSARY

**epistemology:** a philosophical standpoint onto the research process that asks such questions as, What can we know and who can know? A researcher's epistemology encompasses her/his standpoint on the nature of knowledge and learning.

**interpretative approach:** has the specific core assumption that reality is socially constructed and focuses on understanding the meaning of social reality from the perspective of the individual's experiences. There is an underlying philosophical concern with meaning and how social actors give meaning to their social interactions. The goal of this approach is to ascertain these meanings and, through this subjective understanding, to gain knowledge of the social world. This approach is not necessarily critical of the social structures that social actors inhabit, nor is there necessarily a social transformation/social change goal, as in, for example, critical theory, postmodern, or feminist perspectives.

**nested or embedded design:** a mixed methods design whereby both the qualitative and quantitative data are collected concurrently with one dataset labeled primary and the other secondary. Each dataset answers a different question and/or is collected and analyzed at a different level of analysis (i.e., one at the "macro" level and one at the "micro" level).

**ontology:** a philosophical standpoint onto the research process that asks such questions as, What is the nature of reality? Ontologies are theories on the nature of being and existence.

**positivism:** employs logical and objective methods (mainly quantitative) and embraces a rational, detached approach to getting at knowledge, with the goal of discerning patterns of social behavior in order to ascertain "laws of human behavior."

**purposive sample:** a collection of specific informants whom a researcher deems likely to exemplify patterns that he or she seeks to pursue in an in-depth qualitative study.

## DISCUSSION QUESTIONS

**1.** How do qualitative and quantitative approaches to research differ?

**2.** How do some researchers use a secondary quantitative study first, followed by the primary qualitative study?

**3.** Why do qualitative researchers use mixed methods designs?

**4.** What are the challenges of a mixed methods research design from a qualitative perspective?

## ■ ■ ■ SUGGESTED WEBSITES ■ ■ ■

*www.colorado.edu/journalism/mcm/qmr-const-theory.htm*

A professor and researcher of media and culture describes her definitions and arguments for qualitative research and constructivism.

*www.colorado.edu/journalism/mcm/qmr-crit-theory.htm*

The same researcher as in the preceding entry discusses critical theory.

## NOTES

1. The whole idea of primary and secondary components of a mixed methods project can become a confusing issue. Both components are essential, and sometimes the use of these terms and their notation (i.e., quan, QUAN, qual, QUAL) is not useful. What is important to focus on is how both components play a role in answering the research question.

2. Excerpts from Mactavish and Schleien (2004). Copyright 2004 by John Wiley & Sons Ltd. Reprinted by permission.

3. A gender-comparison component was not possible for the baby-boomer generation study, due to the small number of women physicians practicing at the time.

# CHAPTER 5

# Feminist Approaches to Mixed Methods Research

Feminist perspectives of the social world embody a variety of different standpoints and outlooks, but all are concerned with creating a more socially just world, especially for women and other oppressed groups. The purposes of this chapter are to illuminate feminist perspectives on social science research and to provide examples of how feminist researchers use a qualitative approach to mixed methods in order to problematize, advance our understanding of, and even create social change around the issue of gender inequality.

## What Is Feminist Research?

Qualitative methods have long been associated with feminist research. Feminist researchers debate the appropriateness of different methods in studying women's lives (Bowles & Duelli Klein, 1983; Roberts, 1981). Some researchers argue that only qualitative methods can capture the subtleties and nuances of women's lived experiences and, furthermore, that these methods are "better" and "more feminist" than quantitative approaches (Miner-Rubino & Jayaratne, 2007, p. 300). Indeed, some feminist researchers claim that quantitative methods reinforce the status quo by operating from within an androcentric positivist paradigm (Harding, 1991, 1993; Hartsock, 1998; Reinharz, 1992; Smith, 1987a).

This chapter argues that feminist methods are fluid and that there is not one set of methods that are distinctly feminist. From our perspective, methods are tools or techniques researchers employ in order to answer specific research questions; they are not inherently feminist or nonfeminist. What makes feminist research "feminist" lies in the perspectives and research questions that focus on the lives of women. Feminist research probes questions of power, difference, silence, and oppression, with the goal of moving toward a more just society for women and other oppressed groups. Feminist researchers study women's issues by listening to their voices, exploring and thus empowering their experiences, and examining connections between power and knowledge.

Criticism of the positivist paradigm has prompted a considerable amount of research by feminists. During the 1970s and 1980s, *feminist empiricists,* those feminist researchers who worked from within a positivist tradition, worked to "deconstruct" what they perceived as errors within their disciplines after discovering that male biases in science cascaded across fields such as psychology, philosophy, history, sociology, education, anthropology, and language and communications (Harding, 1987, 1998). These feminist researchers set out with the goal of eradicating sexist research. A fundamental argument of these feminist researchers was that women were "left out" of existing knowledge and that their issues, needs, and concerns needed to be included in research endeavors.

Other feminist researchers, such as Sprague and Zimmerman (2004) and Nielsen (1990), challenged the viability of generally accepted concepts in positivism, such as objectivity and universality, that require the researcher to maintain a value-free and detached stance from his or her research project. Also, the creation of false dichotomies such as the "subject–object" split serve to bias the research process. Hesse-Biber and Yaiser (2004) write:

> Positivist science assumes a subject–object split where the researcher is taken for granted as the knowing party. The researcher and researched, or, knower and knowable, are on different planes within the research process. By privileging the researcher as the knowing party a hierarchy paralleling that of patriarchal culture is reproduced. Unequal power relations between the research and research participants serve to transform the research subject into an object. . . . Positivists traditionally *seek* knowledge in a narrow self-contained way whereas feminists aim at *developing* knowledge with their research

subjects who bring their own experiential knowledge, concern, and emotions to the project. (p. 12)

Positivist research has also served to marginalize and exclude women, minorities, and other groups from its research for decades, all under the guise of scientific neutrality. Positivism has been linked with social dominance in several ways:

(1) the conduct of research is carried out through social relationships of differential power with the attendant risks of exploitation and abuse; (2) research is inherently political in facilitating particular structures of power within the larger society, either those already in existence or those through which the currently oppressed are empowered. (Sprague & Zimmerman, 1993, quoted in Hesse-Biber & Yaiser, 2004, p. 13)

Alternately, some feminist researchers, such as Donna Haraway (1988), Kum-Kum Bhavnani (1993), and Sandra Harding (1987), argue for a *feminist objectivity*. Haraway defines this type of objectivity as "situated knowledge," promoting the idea that knowledge and truth are partial, situated, subjective, power imbued, and relational. Denying the existence of values, biases, and politics in research is undesirable, and these feminist researchers assert that more objective knowledge is achieved or accessed by acknowledging the specificity and unique aspects of the researchers' and the research participants' social positioning and experiences.

Feminist researchers have also introduced other knowledge-building models that are rooted in research about women's lives. *Feminist standpoint theory* considers women's everyday experiences while analyzing the gaps that can occur when women work to fit themselves into the general culture's way of understanding women's positionality. It acknowledges that the oppressed (in this case, women) exist in a dualistic space, living through two perspectives; their personal perspective and the perspective of their oppressors, to whom they adapt (Hesse-Biber & Yaiser, 2004, p. 15). According to Nancy Hartsock (1983), this enables women to "have greater insight as researchers into the lives of other women" (cited in Hesse-Biber & Yaiser, 2004, p. 15). Feminist standpoint theory also acknowledges the importance of women building knowledge from their own experiences and validates women's individual understanding and lived experiences as foundational for a certain feminist epistemology (Smith, 1987a).

Examining the differences between standpoints assists the researcher in uncovering a more accurate explanation of the lives of the oppressed and their oppressors. Feminist standpoint epistemology has changed significantly over time, and the notion of *multiple standpoints* considers the interlocking relationships that link racism, sexism, heterosexism, and class oppression in our social reality (Collins, 2000; Higginbotham, 1992; hooks, 1989, 1990, 1992; Reay, 1998; Weber, 1998; Weston & Rofel, 1984). This understanding is deeply ingrained in the concept of feminist research.

Feminist researchers engage with issues of difference in many fields. Studying intersections between gender, race, ethnicity, and class has expanded feminist researchers' focus on issues of difference; issues of sexual preference, disability, and nationality have also deepened the understanding of difference. Feminist scholars are increasingly aware of a need to examine global issues facing women and have placed particular emphasis on imperialism, colonialism, and national identity in this framework. The following factors sum up our discussion of the basic essence of what feminist research encompasses:

- Feminist researchers ask new questions. Feminist research stresses the need to explore women's subjugated knowledge by giving voice to women's experiences. In particular, the focus is on knowledge that traditional research approaches have marginalized, often leaving out gender as a category of inquiry.

- Feminist research stresses the importance of getting at multiple understandings of the nature of social reality, particularly as this pertains to women's concerns and standpoints.

- Feminist researchers address issues of difference. Feminist research advocates for the importance of studying across differences in terms of gender, race, class, and so on.

- Feminist research stresses the importance of the empowerment of women in the research process by advocating the practice of *reflexivity*, which calls forth an awareness of power imbalances between the researcher and the researched, the need to be mindful of the research concepts used within a given study, and the importance of listening throughout the research process.

- Feminist research stresses the importance of social justice, social transformation, and social change on behalf of women and other oppressed groups.

## Mixed Methods and the Feminist Approach

This chapter presents in-depth case studies showing why and how feminists use mixed methods research. Some feminists might choose mixed methods for the same reasons that nonfeminist researchers do, but some feminists' reasons for employing mixed methods are based on the nature of the specific research questions they seek to answer. Although feminists' interests cross all epistemological boundaries, there are particular nuances and concerns that go into shaping feminist methodologies regardless of their epistemological assumptions.

With mixed methods research, then, the possibility exists for researchers to apply a range of methods to assist them in seeking out subjugated knowledge that dominant perspectives on knowledge building often miss (Reinharz, 1992). More specifically, the practice of mixed methods holds open the possibility of increasing the layers of meaning that often remain subjugated and undifferentiated by using a range of different types of methods in the service of women's issues and concerns. The addition of quantitative methods to a qualitative approach also provides a mechanism for legitimating women's knowledge building by testing out new theories, as well as placing women's lived experience in a broader sociopolitical context. This dual-methods approach is also an effective strategy to advance social policy and to promote social change for women.

Mixed methods research provides feminists with a strategy for responding to traditional forms of knowledge building, particularly as it pertains to standard research measures such as those that appear in quantitative survey research. For example, standard measures of economic activity such as "work" have often reflected only paid employment. Underneath this measure is a set of assumptions concerning the role of men and women in society; restricting the definition of work to paid employment neglects a range of unpaid economic activity, including the majority of work done by women, especially in developing societies in which women engage in subsistence activities such as farming. By pushing on the boundaries of traditional economic measures, feminist researchers bring a new perspective to the meaning of work that includes both paid and unpaid labor (Hesse-Biber & Carter, 2005). Using quantitative measures in tandem with qualitative methods provides a mechanism for changing the ways in which research is practiced.

Multiple objectives are often contained within any given feminist research project. This chapter explores how feminist researchers tackle some of these major dimensions of feminist research by presenting some in-depth examples of how mixed methods can serve to further feminist research goals. It is clear, however, that feminist goals mentioned earlier often overlap with other qualitative approaches. For example, qualitative approaches such as a transformative qualitative approach (Mertens, 2005) focus on social justice and social change. Critical and postmodern qualitative approaches stress the power dynamics in the knowledge-building process and seek to uncover dominant forms of knowledge with the goal of deconstructing knowledge that is taken as the "truth." A feminist perspective emphasizes the importance of centering women's concerns as the subject of inquiry and being mindful of how women's standpoints also differ in terms of such factors as race, ethnicity, class, and sexual preference.

## Using a Feminist Mixed Methods Approach to Reveal Subjugated Knowledge and Silenced Voices

Mixed methods research offers feminists the opportunity to uncover subjugated knowledge and silenced voices. Feminist researchers often start out their research projects by employing a qualitative method or methods. By initiating a qualitative method, they might pragmatically build quantitative measures into their research design or dialectically integrate the two sides of their research methods in a balanced and integrated approach.

### Case Study 1: Understanding Land Forest Usage in Nepal

We start with a case study that employs an integrated mixed methods approach, balanced in that both qualitative and quantitative methods occupy an equal footing, with both methods informing one another at the analysis and interpretation stages.

Andrea Nightingale is a feminist geographer who is interested in community land forest usage in Mugu, Nepal. Her general research agenda is to understand how different actors, including the state, communities, and international donors within community forestry, experience different types of knowledge about the forest. She takes an overall relational approach to forest usage in that she views the forest not only as a physical entity but also as a sociocultural environment that interacts with the forest's "natural" environment. She put it this way:

Studies of community forestry assume first and foremost the presence of a forest and yet taking a more relational perspective demands
that the processes that produce a "forest" (materially, symbolically,
politically) are explained. . . . How is it that community forests are
sustained as "forests"? . . . It is not simply the details of management,
ecological conditions and contestations over knowledge that are significant, but also how these aspects of forests are produced, framed,
(re)told and therefore brought into view that are important. . . . The
specific ecological processes of water and soil movement, seedling
establishment and tree growth are only sustained in that configu-
ration by harvesting practices, management strategies and political
relationships. One does not pre-exist the other and cannot be understood in isolation. . . . (Nightingale, 2006b)

Using a feminist standpoint perspective, this particular case study
examines this research question: What is the lived experience of different women with regard to community forestry usage?[1]

To uncover women's lived experiences regarding community forestry usage, Nightingale employs a feminist standpoint perspective
that relies on Donna Haraway's (1988) concept that all knowledge is
situationally based. Unlike those researchers who embrace a positivist
paradigm, the feminist epistemological conception of social reality that
Haraway employs assumes that all knowledge is partial, value laden,
and context bound. Correspondingly, the denial of values, biases, and
politics is problematic, leading to a replication of dominant cultural
understandings of a given social phenomenon. Haraway (1988) defines
feminist objectivity as *situated knowledges*, meaning that it acknowledges
how and from what standpoint or context knowledge has been produced.

Nightingale (2003) pointed out that, prior to the 1990s, feminist
geographers were "feminist empiricists" whose primary goal was to
eradicate sexist research by simply including women in their research
projects. However, locating gender differences in their analysis and
interpretation of their research findings was not necessarily the focus
of their research. In contrast, Nightingale's feminist standpoint epistemology places women's issues as a *central point of inquiry* in terms of the
questions asked, the data gathered, and the analysis and interpretation of land forest usage. It was from this *standpoint epistemology* that she
developed a series of research questions that stress the importance of
understanding the experiences of women and other oppressed groups
regarding forest use. She noted:

In my own work on community forestry in Nepal, I used qualitative, ethnographic techniques, such as oral histories, participant–observation and in-depth interviewing, as well as aerial photo interpretation and quantitative vegetation inventory. In addition to highlighting the situatedness and partiality of knowledge, the Nepali case study also helps to show the importance of challenging "dominant" representations of forest change—in this case aerial photo interpretation—not by rejecting them outright, but by demonstrating explicitly how they provide only one part of the story of forest change. This is a particularly important project in Nepal where increasingly remote sensed data are used to determine changes in forest cover, land use and environmental degradation. (Nightingale, 2003, p. 80)

Nightingale (2003) employed a mixed methods research design to explore the silenced or unexplored voices of women from different caste rankings by gathering multiple types of data: oral histories of women, official documents, and aerial photos of the forest landscape utilizing global positioning systems (GPS). The combined usage of qualitative and quantitative methods allowed her to uncover women's voices by interrogating discrepancies between her qualitative and quantitative findings. The discrepancies in her findings also demonstrated how knowledge is partial and socially situated. Each type of data collected is an important aspect of forest usage but from a different knowledge standpoint. Using GPS data alone as primary evidence of forest usage, as practiced by traditional geographic researchers, provides only a partial view of forest usage. Nightingale (2003) also noted that traditional geographers use mixed methods to triangulate their findings; this conventional use of mixed methods, she said, comes from their working from a positivistic standpoint that assumes a unitary view of reality.

This case narrative is also about what happens when dominant positivistic methodologies and methods within geography are challenged by new ways of thinking and must deal with the incorporation of qualitative approaches into mixed methods, whose goal is not necessarily to use qualitative data to triangulate with quantitative results. The following excerpt is from an interview conducted with Andrea Nightingale regarding the research project that she began as part of her doctoral dissertation. She began the interview with a story about what happened when she shared her feminist perspective on forest usage with her doctoral committee, as well as what happened when she revealed her decision to use qualitative methods on an equal footing with quantitative

methods in her research design. Let's go behind the scenes with Nightingale as she speaks about her research project.

> *I think I thought that working across the social and natural sciences neces-*
> *sarily entailed using mixed methods. One of the people on my committee*
> *had said to me, "Oh, that would be really interesting because you could use*
> *like aerial interpretations to validate your interviews." And I said, "No, I*
> *don't want to do that because I think that both these forms of knowledge*
> *are valid and I don't want to uphold one over the other." And so it was*
> *more interesting to me to kind of think about well, why were they the same,*
> *or weren't they the same? And what did it mean if they weren't? Not to*
> *sort of say, "Oh well, people must have been lying to me. . . . " I really felt*
> *very strongly that there were different ways of understanding what was*
> *happening with forest change. And I didn't want to privilege one of those*
> *understandings over the other, but rather, I wanted to kind of put them side*
> *by side and see what they said to one another.*

Nightingale's feminist perspective on land usage clashes with the
more dominant geographic perspective that assumes that there is a
"correct" interpretation of forest usage and that to obtain an interpretation of land cover and land forms researchers should cross-check areas
on each photo with areas on the ground. Yet this simple method of
comparison raised a central question for Nightingale's research: Do the
interviews and the photos tell the same story?

Using a feminist standpoint perspective, Nightingale set out to
answer her research question about how women use the forest. She
employed ethnographic techniques, more specifically ecological oral
histories and field observations, asking women to relate their past and
present perceptions of land forest usage and their assessment of ecological conditions of the forest environment. These narratives formed
snapshots of women's experiences, allowing a linking of present and
past experiences.

She also conducted an aerial photo analysis, a quantitative approach
used by traditional geographers to systematically categorize forest
land—its textures, colors, and shades within the photos. She conducted
a quantitative content analysis of aerial photos of the forest area from
both 1978 and 1996 by mapping landscape changes in the forest.

Nightingale displayed some trepidation concerning her mixed
methods design, especially with regard to challenging some members
of her doctoral committee who do not share her feminist approach

to knowledge building and who in fact might expect her to use her qualitative oral histories as a "check" (or form of triangulation) on her quantitative aerial photo analysis. However, would the lived experiences of those who use the land over time match what she discovered in her quantitative aerial photo analysis? What would a discrepancy between her oral histories and aerial photo interpretation reveal about how land forest usage is interpreted using a traditional quantitative approach versus a feminist standpoint approach that privileges the voices of women?

A feminist standpoint approach to land forest usage allows Nightingale not just to see nature as something in an aerial photo but also to look at the nature–society boundary. Nature is also socially and physically constructed by society in the basic interactions of the individual with the natural landscape. Nightingale's mixed methods feminist approach reveals new conceptual space to rethink the nature–society interface. What is hidden in the aerial photos of the forest is a set of societal gendered relationships.

Not only did Nightingale mix methods at the data collection phase of her research, but she also mixed data analysis techniques. The quantitative and qualitative analyses were treated equally, and both types of findings were interwoven into her analysis. She used one type of data to inform the other. She compared different types of research findings and did not necessarily expect them to agree (triangulate). Both data-sets were equally important, and one did not preempt the other. She commented:

> A different research design might have used photos merely to set the context for forest change and then used the histories to detail the cultural and political aspects of that change. Instead, by setting the datasets in relation to each other I have allowed for both to be acknowledged as partial and situated. (Nightingale, 2003, p. 86)

Andrea Nightingale's feminist approach to mixed methods research revealed that aerial photo analysis alone did not provide a complete understanding of the process of land forest usage. The qualitative component of the mixed methods design uncovered women's pivotal role in land forest usage and the importance of taking into account the networks of gendered social relations in understanding the forest landscape and its transformation over time.[2] In particular, Nightingale sought to look at the ways in which "forest management regimes" serve to promote gender inequality (looking at differences between women by caste, as well as ethnicity) by privileging men's access to resources and control over community forestry and management. As a result of her research, she brought previously unexplored and unresearched voices of women into hearing, and the use of mixed methods allowed this.

### Case Study 2: Uncovering the Silenced Sexual Desire of Adolescent Girls

We turn to another case study that shows how combining mixed methods at the data analysis stage can also serve to uncover subjugated knowledge—in this case, young girls' experiences of their sexuality. Girls' knowledge of sexuality oftentimes relies on sex education in the school system. Deborah L. Tolman and Laura A. Szalacha (1999) applied a mixed methods design to the study of adolescent girls' sexuality and their experiences of sexual desire. Girls formally receive information about sex from their school's sex education programs, but many of these are devoid of information dealing with sexual desire.

Tolman and Szalacha (1999) sought to uncover how girls talk about their sexuality, especially as this pertains to sexual desires. Michelle Fine (1988) noted that there is a "missing discourse of desire" in these sex education programs for adolescents and in society in general, causing the topic of sexual desire to become taboo and making it hard for adolescents in general and girls in particular to find a space to reflect on their own sexuality and feel a sense of agency about their own sexual practices. In other words, girls do not have a language with which to speak about their own feelings of desire. Tolman and Szalacha's (1999) work centered on the concerns of adolescent girls in their research practice, with the goal of uncovering this "missing discourse of desire" (Fine, 1988, p. 31). They wanted to know (1) How do adolescent girls talk about their experiences of sexuality? (2) How do they respond to their own sense of sexual desire?

They collected both quantitative and qualitative data simultaneously by administering a standard set of survey questions followed by open-ended interview questions. These follow-up questions were guided by a "feminist relational approach" that used each interviewee's closed-ended responses to guide the construction of qualitative questions in a second part of the study (Tolman & Szalacha, 1999, p. 13); in this phase, girls' specific and unique experiences and their feelings of sexual desire were explored.

Tolman and Szalacha's (1999) research also employed a mixed methods analysis of their data, whereby their entire dataset was contextualized and recontextualized in order to get micro patterns (understanding individual adolescents' sexual desires), as well as macro patterns (by grouping these individual accounts in order to discern any specific patterns or differences across urban and suburban groups), within their data.

The first part of their mixed methods analysis was the qualitative component. They analyzed the individual voices of 30 girls and looked for specific themes within their data. They employed a narrative "listening guide" that was designed to pick up "the variety of multi-layered voices that often co-exist within a person's narrative" (see Brown & Gilligan, 1992, p. 21). In their analysis of these data, they came up with four voices involved in girls' experiences of sexual desire: a "voice of the self, an erotic voice, a voice of the body, and a voice of response to one's own desire" (Tolman & Szalacha, 1999, p. 14). The results of their findings led the researchers to perform a more quantitative analysis, and they recontextualized their data by changing the unit of analysis from the individual female to the "narrative." This shifted the focus from intensive interviews with 30 girls to an analysis of the numerous types of narratives found among the 30 girls as a whole. This process yielded 128 narratives, enough individual data points to allow a statistical analysis of their qualitative data.

These narratives were analyzed quantitatively by classifying them into urban and suburban narratives (depending on where the girls lived). The authors wanted to explore themes of vulnerability and pleasure, but they also sought to examine "how pleasure and vulnerability were associated differently for these two groups of girls . . . [and] whether there was an interactive effect of sexual abuse or violence" (Tolman & Szalacha, 1999, p. 17).

They applied an in-depth analysis to the narratives of both suburban and urban groups. The researchers searched for differences within and between the groups regarding themes of pleasure and vulnerability. They then searched for a possible relationship between these two narrative themes and the narrator's geographic location. They noted some important relationships within and between these groups of narratives, stating:

We are also able to highlight that an interplay between these girls' social locations and personal histories of sexual violation figures significantly in how they experience and give meaning to their own desire, specifically pinpointing how they are limited and supported in the possibility of associating their own sexual desire with pleasure. (Tolman & Szalacha, 1999, p. 21)

Although Tolman and Szalacha (1999) found modest differences between the narratives of urban and suburban girls regarding vulnerability with regard to sexual desire, once they controlled for the presence or absence of sexual abuse, this difference disappeared. They did find a larger difference in expressions of sexual pleasure among suburban girls' experiences compared with the urban group's narratives. It was found that urban girls, in this study, "make a conscious choice to sacrifice pleasure to protect themselves from danger," an issue that did not come up in interviews with the suburban girls (pp. 16–17).

A mixed methods analysis approach to their data allowed Tolman and Szalacha to bring voice and experience to the study of adolescent females' sexuality. Recontextualizing their analysis using a quantitative analytical approach allowed them to see the patterns within their data and, within these categories, to apply qualitative analytical techniques to uncover further important differences among urban and suburban narratives. This set of mixed analytical methods enabled them to tease out the many differences found among adolescent girls' stories and, furthermore, to reinterpret and reconcile the inconsistencies in the data instead of dismissing results that seemed contradictory. These analytical procedures enabled communication between methods. Their analysis of the qualitative data revealed a distinction between urban versus suburban girls. Urban girls were more concerned about the risky consequences of experiencing their sexual desire, as articulated in themes of danger and vulnerability in their narratives (e.g., risks of pregnancy, sexual victimization, and sexually transmitted diseases [STDs]). In contrast, suburban girls experienced anxiety about their sexual desire in terms of what it might reflect about them or how others might perceive them in light of the sexual double standard and its mandate for women to conceal or mute their expressions of sexual desire. This dynamic was reflected in statements such as the following: "I don't like to think of myself as feeling really sexual" (Tolman & Szalacha, 1999, p. 16).

The studies by Andrea Nightingale and by Tolman and Szalacha underscore the importance of a mixed methods design in making subjugated knowledge visible. What makes a feminist mixed methods design important here is that it is especially engaged with women's voices and subjective experiences, and it is in this context that the researchers employ both qualitative and quantitative methods in the service of revealing women's voices. In addition to liberating women's voices, the researchers seek to empower and promote social transformation for women. A feminist perspective on mixed methods seeks to highlight women's issues and bring into focus how institutions may negatively affect women's lives.

## Using a Feminist Mixed Methods Approach to Understand Differences among Women

Patricia Hill Collins's (2000) work argues for understanding differences among women and between women and men within a "matrix of domination" in a way that elucidates the differences among individuals by considering a range of interlocking inequalities in terms of race, class, and gender (p. 228). Depending on his or her social location—that is, social location within these social structures of race, class, gender, and sexuality—any given individual's experience may differ. These social constructs and the institutionalized inequalities or privileges that result from them can limit, as well as broaden, the experiences of both men and women, and it is thus important to remember to include these elements in research in order to create a more far-reaching understanding of individuals' experiences. The following case study looks at the experience of college through the lens of both gender and race.

### Case Study 3: Understanding Complexity in Racial and Gender Identity among African American College Women

In her article "The Influence of Both Race and Gender on the Experiences of African American College Women," Lisa Jackson (1998) explores the interconnections between race and gender in the lives of African American college students. Jackson challenges the practice of research that focuses only on race or gender. Jackson wanted to understand how college-age African American women "define their identity in terms of both race and gender" (1998, p. 360). She addressed the following two questions (p. 362): (1) What is the relationship between race and gender within the self-concept of African American college women? (2) How are the race and gender identities of African American women shaped by the race and gender composition of the colleges they attend?

Jackson (1998) sought to answer this question using a mixed methods design for the purpose of complementarity (p. 362). She argued for the use of both qualitative and quantitative methods when she noted that the "results from one method type are intended to enhance, illustrate, or clarify results from the other" (p. 362). In her study, her qualitative methods informed her quantitative methods.

Her sample consisted of 135 African American women from four colleges. Two samples were from "historically Black" colleges, and the other two were from "predominantly White colleges or universities." Two of the colleges were coeducational, whereas the other two were women's colleges. The study had the following research design.

Jackson (1998) conducted a two-phase mixed methods explanatory design that implemented quantitative and qualitative methods in a sequence. She initially collected quantitative data with questionnaires to be numerically analyzed. She then used these data to select participants for the in-depth interview element of the study. These qualitative interviews helped explain the quantitative results. Within this design, it appears that the quantitative component was primary and the qualitative component was secondary.

The quantitative component consisted of a series of questions on demographic information, as well as standardized tests that measured the ways in which participants answered the question, "Who am I?" Jackson specifically focused on instances in which respondents indicated race, gender, or race and gender together as the first answer to the question, "Who am I?" Jackson calculated the numbers of women at each school who thought about racial and gender identities as separate, and she discovered that women at almost all of the schools thought about these identities as unified wholes rather than as disconnected aspects of themselves (1998, p. 363). The qualitative component consisted of interviews with those respondents who agreed to a follow-up interview, selected from the range of college environments. Jackson wanted to explore how African American women negotiated their identities within different racial and gender environments.

Jackson's qualitative findings revealed how "race and gender are important and related constructs within the self-concept of African American women" (1998, p. 370). The qualitative data revealed themes of struggle and consciousness relating to the idea of being an African American woman. Her in-depth analysis of women's experiences across the different school environments revealed that a college's racial and gender composition had an important impact on African American women's racial and social identities. Students attending predominantly white colleges experienced the pressure of "proving themselves" to white students and faculty, and at all of the schools studied in Jackson's sample, "African American women struggle to not lose a connection with their racial/ethnic community while simultaneously they strive for success and recognition in the larger society" (1998, p. 370). Whereas the quantitative portion of Jackson's study revealed the extent to which women experience race and gender as interconnected parts of their identities, the subsequent qualitative study revealed the processes by which women constructed their multifaceted sense of self and the impact of varied social environments on these processes. Jackson's study highlights the manner in which qualitative and quantitative methods can be used to complement each other and thereby deepen and complexify an inquiry into the interconnections among gender, race, and class in women's lives.

## Using a Feminist Mixed Methods Approach to Empower Women's Lives

Feminist researchers are mindful of the power imbalances in the research process and seek to understand the meaning of quantitative results within the larger context of women's lives; they do so with the goal of empowering women's voices within the research process and beyond. The next case study reflects this concern and suggests that the deployment of survey findings—especially as they pertain to women's medical treatment—without understanding how they affect individual women's lives can serve to disempower women's concerns and experiences.

### Case Study 4: Empowering Women's Voices in the Study of Postpartum Depression

Feminist psychologist Paula Nicholson (2004) is interested in how women experience postpartum depression. She noted that most of the research in the area of postpartum depression employs clinical trials that seek to specifically measure the effectiveness of certain antidepressant drugs by randomizing respondents into categories—usually a control group (that does not get the drug), an experimental group (that gets the drug), and a placebo group (that receives a "fake drug"). This research method is widely accepted as the "gold standard" for measuring the efficacy of certain medications and is the preferred method to receive funding by the federal government or drug companies.

Nicholson's research took a feminist psychological approach to the issue of postpartum depression and, in doing so, advocated for a mixed methods design that combines clinical research trial (CRT) quantitative data with qualitative data that places an emphasis on contextualizing the quantitative findings through understanding the lived experiences of mothers with postpartum depression. She noted that without the addition of a qualitative component to these studies, there is a tendency for clinicians "to pathologize the female body and mind, paying no regard to women's experiences" (p. 210).

Nicholson (2004) mixed CRT quantitative methods with a longitudinal 6-month qualitative pilot study of 17 women who took part in a CRT. She conducted in-depth interviews with women with postpartum depression four times during a 6-month period, starting after their delivery. Her pilot study revealed that a mixed methods approach, in this case a qualitative study conducted after a quantitative study, provides researchers with a rich understanding of the effectiveness of medication for treating postpartum depression from the perspective of women undergoing treatment. She noted that "although behavior and mood might be similar at three and six months after the birth, the construction and meaning of the experiences are different" (p. 224).

A qualitative component also provides a context for the researcher's results. For example, the quantitative finding that a "poor marital relationship" is highly related to postpartum depression can gain complexity, meaning, and further elucidation by using in-depth interviews to explore what such a marital situation means in the context of a given mother's family life. In addition, the researchers have an opportunity to understand the extent to which respondents evaluate a specific drug intervention, as well as how they evaluate the entire research experience itself, providing the researchers with valuable information that will "lead to more effective intervention and preventative measures" for postpartum depression (2004, p. 220).

The goal of a mixed methods design, then, is not only to elaborate on the findings from the clinical trial data but also to provide a rich context from which clinicians can understand and treat women's specific concerns and issues with regard to postpartum depression. The qualitative findings open up space to empower women's voices and reframe clinical findings and interpretations.

# Using a Feminist Mixed Methods Approach
# for Social Change
# and Social Policy Transformation

Feminist research aims for social transformation and change for women and other oppressed groups. Feminists often employ their research findings in the service of public policy issues. Bringing these issues into an academic and public arena helps publicize the stories and oppressed voices of certain social groups and can spawn societal change and policy initiatives through its publication.

### Case Study 5: Using Research to Change the Status of Women in the Forestry Industry

Maureen G. Reed, a feminist geographer, is interested in women's experiences working in male-dominated occupations in rural forestry communities in British Columbia. She notes that research in this area and government forestry policies neglect or consider women's work and community contributions as peripheral to forestry work. Forestry work conjures up images of logging, an occupation characterized by hard physical labor, danger, and an overall general rough-and-tumble life. Government policy echoes these sentiments, as she noted:

> Women were considered part of forestry communities only when they were attached as partners to male workers who were considered the dominant breadwinners. In 1994, the Commission on Resources and Environment (CORE) reported that "on Vancouver Island about 95% of resource workers are male, and about 80% of them are married. . . . In this statement, CORE only considered women by their conjugal status and recognised only one possible status. Furthermore, CORE neglected that women themselves might be forestry workers with insights and experiences relevant to the changing employment conditions for forestry workers. (Reed, 2003a, p. 373)

The mid-1990s were an especially important time, as the forestry industry in Canada was undergoing structural change in land management (moving from old growth to second growth of timber, dealing with overcutting and lack of adequate tree-renewal policies, and shifting to new governmental forestry protection policies), as well as dealing with issues of land allocation, especially regarding the rights of aboriginal First Nations people. Governmental policies also began to change the nature of forest work, as logging decreased and jobs in forest management increased with a newly emerging demand for forest cultivation and planning. This transition from heavy labor to management opened the door for women's employment in forestry, and Reed started her research at this critical juncture of change in forestry work.

As a feminist and social activist geographer, Reed wanted to unearth the subjugated experiences of women in forestry communities undergoing transition. She wrote:

> I believe that the voices of women have been muted within the institutions that shape public policy making and that their stories are legitimate ones. My interest in activism is strategic. I deliberately go beyond the front lines of political protest and enter the communities, the homes, and the personal lives of forestry-town women whose stories have yet to be told. (Reed, 2003b, p. x)[3]

Her specific research problem in this case study illustration focused on women employed in the forestry industry. Her general research question was: How do women experience living in forestry communities undergoing transition?

In order to understand women's experiences, Reed employed a mixed methods approach to data collection and analysis. She gathered quantitative data in the form of content analysis of public policy documents and examined census track data to unearth a demographic profile of women's overall employment in forestry occupations in the nine forestry communities in Vancouver, British Columbia. The use of quantitative census data enhanced the generalizability of Reed's research in that these data on the entire region selected for her study provided a point of comparison with her subsample of 50 women. She noted that, in fact, her sample had "higher rates of university education and labour force participation and lower rates of unemployment [than those in the region of the study population]" (2003a, p. 376).

She and her staff collected primary data from 37 in-depth interviews with women in forestry and conducted three focus groups with women who lived and worked in the nine forestry communities in her study. She employed a *feminist participatory action research model* for this segment of her study by selecting and training 10 female community researchers who collected additional in-depth interviews with local women in forestry and who were part of three focus groups, providing her with feedback on her analysis by "corroborating and refining emerging themes and social categories" (2003b, p. 21). A second layer of action research participation consisted of workshops she held within the community as a whole. These workshops provided her with additional opportunities for refining her data analysis.

Reed's overall mixed methods research represents more of an *interactive mixed model* in that she iteratively collects data, analyzes it, collects more data, and so on. There does not appear to be a specific sequencing of qualitative and quantitative methods wherein one method is primary and the other secondary or in which the stress is on the importance of ordering methods in a sequential or concurrent manner, as exhibited in the mixed methods designs highlighted in Chapter 2. Instead, methods are employed in the service of answering questions guided by a feminist epistemology that seeks to unearth women's marginalized experiences working in the male-dominated forestry industry—an industry that renders them invisible to policy makers, academics, and government agencies.

Reed's iterative deployment of mixed methods allowed her to integrate the findings from one method with the findings from another in a "back and forth" motion of information flow and analysis, making it difficult to categorize her research as a specific mixed methods design. For example, in gathering census track data, Reed noticed that the occupational categories reflected male-dominated cultures, leading to an undercount of women's actual contributions to forestry work. The occupational categories were designed to reflect "men in forestry occupations," often excluding specific occupational categories, such as office jobs, in which women are in fact employed in forestry work (2003b, p. 103). Reed's data from in-depth interviews allowed her to question census definitions of occupational categories by suggesting the need for refinement of these categories in order to reflect women's occupational lives.

As Hesse-Biber and Yaiser (2004) note, one aspect of feminist research is to "seek methods that empower their respondents and participants as well as their research" (p. 277). By questioning census category data, Reed showed awareness of how categories of measurement can render invisible women's contributions to the forestry industry. Her use of findings from her qualitative data provided her with new ways to unearth the marginalized perspectives of women and to address their needs and concerns. At the same time, her work challenges the androcentrism of the official census occupational categories, opening up the possibility for a more equitable measurement of women's labor force contributions to the forestry industry as a whole.

Reed's inclusion of in-depth focus groups allowed an integration of the lived experience of women into the analysis of the in-depth qualitative data. The focus-group research provided her with ways to refine her analysis and to ask new questions concerning her research problem, as well as her interpretation of research findings. In-depth analysis of her qualitative data also served to inform her research question and the underlying theoretical perspectives that informed her research. Reed noted that early feminist literature painted an either/or view of women in forestry: liberal interpretations saw them as victims, and socialist interpretations saw their participation in the male-dominated workforce as victory over their powerless social, economic, and political situation.

The findings gathered from Reed's mixed methods data collection and analysis had a dramatic impact on her initial theoretical ideas on employed women's roles in male-dominated occupations. Instead of revealing a clear-cut answer to her alternative theoretical models on women in forestry, she found a dramatic paradox contained within her qualitative data: employed women both supported and challenged patriarchal cultural practices in their workplace and in their community. She demonstrated the importance of taking into account women's "social embeddedness" within their communities in order to understand their contradictory behaviors:

> Women's choices and perspectives about employment are located within systems of social relations and cultural norms that fix their work in particular social and geographic locations. In short, the discourses and practices of women in forestry were socially embedded within local and societal norms and values. Rather, contradictory ideas about inclusion and exclusion, and appropriate feminine and masculine behaviours ran simultaneously within individual interviews and across the discussions with women of differing employment, age and life-stage status. Women's adoption of cultural norms and values associated with forestry reflected and reinforced their own marginality. Women are both social activists against patriarchal norms and at the same time compliant with some aspects of these norms. (Reed, 2003a, p. 387)

It is this dual understanding of how women are embedded socially and occupationally within their communities that allowed Reed to understand, first, how they simultaneously participated in their own subjugation while actively challenging their oppressed position and, second, how the interaction of these two forces continues to keep them at the margins of the forestry industry:

> The binary of victim/victor does not grant sufficient attention to the complexity and contradiction that characterize women's lives and

perspectives. Rather, I suggest that through discourse and practice, women are co-creators of the forestry culture and communities that provide openings and closures for women in the paid work of forestry. Greater attention to women's participation in forestry—in practice and in discourse—provides more nuanced theoretical explanations and more accurate empirical descriptions to inform policy choices about forestry employment. (Reed, 2003a, p. 387)

Reed's integration of mixed methods at both the data collection and data analysis stages, especially the deployment of the "participatory action" component (focus groups) of her research, allowed women's work contributions in the forestry industry to become "visible." Such visibility has profound policy implications. Because women's concerns and contributions have been made known through a mixed methods model, women in forestry now have an opportunity to be part of government policy initiatives and have a chance to shape policy debates regarding their own communities. Reed noted that previous government programs focused on retraining or sustaining men in forestry, providing them with resources and retirement packages. Perhaps now they can make these resources available to women workers in the forestry industry.

Reed's mixed methods research also demonstrates the need for women to be more visible in theoretical models that seek to understand structural change in rural societies. Finally, she reminds researchers to practice "reflexivity" in how they deploy their research concepts and to be mindful of the particular biases that can often creep into our measurement tools. Even census categories are not immune to male bias and reflect male-dominated cultures. Reed's data from in-depth interviews allowed her to suggest refinement to quantitative data categories. Her in-depth focus groups and workshop feedback allowed respondents to "talk back" to the qualitative analytical component of her study, providing her with ways to refine her analysis and to provide space for her to reevaluate her initial theoretical lenses and research problem.

## The Need for Mixed Methods Feminist Research Approaches

The case studies we present in this chapter provide a range of examples of how feminists employ mixed methods in the service of feminist research goals, namely, conducting research that uncovers subjugated knowledge and focuses on difference, empowerment, and social change. Feminist researchers are cognizant of the power relationships inherent in any given research project and are especially mindful, through their practices of reflexivity, of their roles as researchers and how the methods they employ may disempower their research respondents. For example, Reed's inclusion of a participatory component in her data gathering and analysis addressed some of the inequalities between her own research position and those of her respondents by selecting respondents to interview their peers.

Feminist researchers employ both qualitative and quantitative methods. What is striking to note in these case studies is the process of mixing methods. The research problem sets the agenda for each study; there is no prior set of fixed mixed methods designs that feminists choose from. Instead, the process of selecting methods is always in conversation with the research goals. The use of a patchwork metaphor as a mode of feminist inquiry is taken from Deleuze and Guattari's (1987) work, in which feminist researchers draw on multiple data sources (patches) and designs (quilt designs), creating space for contradictions and tensions within their research findings, as well as for transformation and social change to occur.

Feminists' practice of using mixed methods often arises in response to findings that crop up during the research process and lead to new questions. Sprague and Zimmerman (2004) comment that when feminist researchers, in efforts to integrate qualitative and quantitative research methods, "encounter apparently different findings from each method . . . [they] need not immediately assume that one should be refuted and the other accepted" (p. 53). We observed this in the case studies conducted by Nightingale and Reed. Such "serendipity" of research findings often allows feminist researchers to clarify or understand disparate results and adds complex meaning to their research. It is in this sense that the process of designing a mixed methods project is iterative; the decision to employ mixed methods design arises "on the fly," depending on prior research findings and whether new questions require the use of a new method. This is not to say, however, that feminist approaches to mixed methods cannot employ mixed methods designs. Some research questions demand a mixed methods design at the outset, whereas other projects may be more serendipitous in their deployment of additional methods. Either way, the researcher's questions always guide the use of a mixed methods model.

Feminists' use of mixed methods as outlined in this chapter is not exhaustive. We address some of the most important characteristics of feminist research that lends itself to a mixed methods approach. As we have stated, feminist research is committed to understanding and addressing the concerns of women and other oppressed groups with a focus on social transformation, social change, and challenging the status quo of scientific knowledge building.

The next chapter addresses postmodern approaches to mixed methods research. This approach, although sharing the common concern of understanding lived experience, does not necessarily center on women's issues and concerns, nor is there necessarily an emphasis on social change and transformation. Postmodern researchers focus their methodological emphasis on the socially constructed nature of the world. The goal of postmodern perspectives is to deconstruct unitary conceptions of truth by uncovering varied and multiple perspectives on social reality and by revealing how discourse shapes our notions of truth, reality, and the social world.

## GLOSSARY

**feminist empiricists:** feminist researchers of the 1970s and 1980s who worked within a positivist tradition to "deconstruct" what they perceived as errors within their disciplines, to eradicate sexist research, and to include women's concerns in research endeavors.

**feminist objectivity:** a type of objectivity in which knowledge and truth are considered partial, situated, subjective, power imbued, and relational.

**feminist standpoint theory:** considers women's everyday experiences while analyzing the gaps that can occur when women work to fit themselves into the general culture's way of understanding women's positionality.

**interactive mixed model:** data collection and analysis occur iteratively with no specific sequencing of qualitative and quantitative methods.

**matrix of domination:** elucidates the differences among individuals by considering a range of interlocking inequalities in terms of race and class, as well as gender.

**situated knowledges:** defined by the context of how and from what standpoint knowledge is produced.

---

### DISCUSSION QUESTIONS

1. How has positivist research worked in opposition to feminist goals?

2. What aspects of feminist research fit well with a mixed methods approach?

3. I say that "mixed methods research offers feminists the opportunity to uncover subjugated knowledge." How is this true? How are women's concerns and contributions made visible by mixed methods research?

---

## ■ ■ ■ SUGGESTED WEBSITES ■ ■ ■

### *Feminist Research*

*www.unb.ca/PAR-L/win/feminmethod.htm*

A definition of what makes feminist research feminist and discussion of qualitative and quantitative methods.

*www.ncrw.org*

The website of the National Council for Research on Women, a network of research, advocacy, and policy centers across the United States.

*plato.stanford.edu/entries/feminism-epistemology/*

*Stanford Encyclopedia of Philosophy* entry on feminist epistemology.

### *Participatory Action Research*

*www.scu.edu.au/schools/gcm/ar/ari/p-ywadsworth98.html*

An in-depth look at participatory action research, which recognizes the social implications of its findings and often actively seeks to study something in order to change or improve it.

## NOTES

1. Nightingale is also interested in several other research goals that we do not take up here, namely, to what extent do women influence decisions over the forest management? Also, what are the implications of the findings from these questions for sustainable resource management over time (Nightingale, 2006a, p. 1)?

2. Although not discussed here, Nightingale also examined how these relations were intertwined and dependent on caste, class, race, and cultural expectations regarding the role of nature and the environment.

3. Excerpt from Reed (2003b). Copyright 2003 by University of British Columbia Press. Reprinted by permission. All rights reserved by the Publisher.

# CHAPTER 6

# Postmodernist Approaches to Mixed Methods Research

with Chris Kelly

Postmodernism and its related schools of thought—poststructuralism (Derrida, 1966), postcolonialism (Mohanty, 1988, 1999; Spivak, 1994), and queer theory (Thomas, 2000), among others—represent an important and rich intellectual heritage that has emerged in the late 20th century. Although these theories and their respective research traditions focus on different aspects of human life and expression, they are all united by the common goal of challenging the status quo of modern enlightenment thought. For the purposes of this chapter, we use "postmodernism" as an umbrella term for these theories, although, as you will see, the term has been and can be used in many different ways. This chapter illuminates the postmodernist perspective and its relevance to social science research and provides examples of how postmodernist researchers have used mixed methods to advance their particular research agendas.

## What Is Postmodernism?

Postmodernist thought emerged in the late 20th century in response to debates in modernist philosophy (between Kant and Hegel and their critics, Nietzsche, the Frankfurt School, and Heidegger), as well as skepticism about the goals and ideals of modern society. Postmodernism, as espoused by the French philosopher Jean-Francois Lyotard (1984) in his book, *The Postmodern Condition: A Report on Knowledge*, represented an active critique of the assumptions of modernity and its promises for a better society that included, most importantly, enlightenment ideas of human progress through scientific advancement and the rational organization of society, as well as notions of the dignity, autonomy, and self-determination of the individual.

Several features that echo throughout postmodern thought are relevant to the social sciences (for a more detailed review of postmodernism, see Agger, 1991; Cheek, 2000; Rosenau, 1992). First, one of the most prominent features of postmodern thought is the rejection of "grand narratives" or "metanarratives." A *metanarrative* is any conceptual system that purports to subsume all of reality within its own universe of meaning, such as Christianity or Marxism (Cheek, 2000). Postmodernists reject the idea that there are objective truths that have universal or transcendental value; instead, they prefer localized, multicultural narratives whose truth value is understood to be partial and even idiosyncratic, grounded as they are in specific cultural contexts and the particular social positioning (i.e., race, class, gender, etc.) of the narrator (Agger, 1991).

Second, whereas *modernism* is premised on a subject or self that is universal, unitary, and autonomous, this assumption is not tenable from a postmodern perspective. Postmodernism challenges the belief in a single subject that is stable over time. Instead, the self or the subject is assumed to be permeable to the outside world. The subject is largely a social or even symbolic construct and is therefore mutable, rather than preexisting (Rosenau, 1992). For this reason, postmodernism tends to advocate altering, if not outright rejecting, the existence of a singular and stable subject in one's analyses and conversely focusing on socially constructed subjectivity with the goal of deconstructing or undoing all constructions of self in order to reveal the underlying contradictions and assumptions that serve to support modernism's totalizing constructions of the self.

Postmodernists also analyze images, symbols, and texts, termed *discourses*, as a window into how social life is constructed and framed by a set of common metanarratives that come to be viewed as "truth." For the postmodernist, knowledge occurs only within and is constructed by discourses (Agger, 1991). Its focus on discourse has made postmodernism a more popular approach in the humanities than in the natural and social sciences. Different varieties of postmodernism share the contention that discourses, defined broadly, play an extremely influential role in how people construe the "real" world. Related to this, knowledge of discourse is inextricably bound up with both the exercise and production of power. As particular dominant discourses (i.e., expert systems of knowledge such as psychiatry or medicine) circulate in society, they come to be viewed as unquestioned, self-evident truths that shape and regulate people's behavior and block from view other discourses that would suggest alternative societal arrangements. Noted by postmodernists as well are the importance of resistance to dominant forms of discourse and the seeking of alternative readings of any given narrative (Foucault, 1975).

Adopting a postmodernist approach necessarily leads a researcher to ask certain types of research questions that are distinctive of the perspective. First, postmodernism does not assume that history is continuous or that society is cohesive but rather emphasizes disruptions, discontinuity, and plurality. This invites questions about contrary and contradictory societal tendencies. Additionally, because the postmodernist subject is constituted through discourse and social experience, questions about the individual are usually questions about that individual's constitution in society and discourse. Indeed, discourses (images, symbols, texts, material practices, etc.), more so than individuals themselves, are likely to be the focus of any social science research that proceeds from a postmodernist paradigm. Lastly, a postmodernist perspective often prompts researchers to ask questions about the nature of power and its relationship to dominant systems of knowledge or discourse in any given social setting.

Postmodernism has many implications for both the methodology (theoretical perspectives) and the methods (tools for collecting and analyzing data) of the social sciences. Postmodernism challenges science's pretensions to objectivity by exposing its class, racial, and gender biases and by arguing in favor of multiple voices, perspectives, and paradigms (Agger, 1991). Additionally, postmodernists question even the most fundamental assumptions of theory and research. Rosenau (1992) argued:

> Post-modernism is oriented towards methods that apply to a broad range of phenomena, focus on the margins, highlight uniqueness, concentrate on the enigmatic, and appreciate the unrepeatable. . . . Post-modern social science presumes methods that multiply paradox . . . rather than methods that settle on solutions. (Rosenau, 1992, p. 117)

Instead of truth claims and metanarratives, postmodernist methods prefer subjective, interpretative approaches that recognize multiple, equally legitimate interpretations. Julianne Cheek (1999) summarized the postmodernist insights on knowledge building, something important to keep in mind as we proceed to apply a postmodern approach to mixed methods research:

> Postmodern approaches provide a challenge to the view that it is possible to represent any aspect of reality in its entirety, speak for others, make truth claims, and attain universal essential understandings. In so doing, postmodern approaches challenge the way that reality has come to be represented. Thus, sometimes postmodern approaches are described as emanating from a crisis in representation. With an emphasis on the plurality of reality, postmodern approaches recognize the multiplicity of voices, views, and methods present in any representation or analysis of any aspect of reality. . . . Such recognition encourage[s] . . . practitioners and researchers to engage in a form of reflexivity, in which the analysis of practice involves multiple layers, multiple truths, and multiple voices. There is no natural or given way to do things or to understand things in a postmodern approach. (Cheek, 1999, p. 385)

## Postmodernist Questions and Mixed Methods Research Design

Postmodernists lie on different points of a continuum with respect to the degree to which they endorse a relativist versus an objectivist (positivist) view of the social reality. Rosenau (1992) provided an important distinction between "skeptical postmodernism" and "affirmative postmodernism" (p. 15). Rosenau noted that *skeptical postmodernism* provides a "pessimistic, negative, [and] gloomy assessment" in which all versions of reality are equally valid and the idea of predicting social reality in any causal way is irrelevant (1992, p. 15). For a skeptical postmodernist, the social world is one of "fragmentation, disintegration, malaise, meaninglessness, a vagueness or even absence of moral parameters and societal chaos" (Rosenau, 1992, p. 15).

On the other hand, an *affirmative postmodernist* is more optimistic and does not buy into the dichotomy of relativism versus objectivism. Instead, there is a dynamic tension that exists between these two ends of the continuum. For example, a feminist postmodernist influenced by an affirmative approach to research inquiry might support knowledge building about women's experiences that is based on women's stand-points as more valid than knowledge building in this area from the standpoint of men. In this instance, a researcher is practicing affirmative postmodernism in that she or he accepts that some versions of reality are truer than others. An affirmative postmodern stance to research can provide an opening up to the subjective aspects of knowledge building and provide a much-needed skepticism in more traditional forms of inquiry such as positivism (Rosenau, 1992).

An example of a skeptical postmodern stance is provided by researchers who work from an "evocative autoethnographic perspective," in which the researchers do not attempt to connect their lived account to any wider theoretical framework or wider set of issues (see Anderson, 2006). Researchers consider different evocative autoethnographic accounts of lived experiences equally plausible and correct.

It is important to note here that a postmodern approach does not exclude the use of quantitative methods. As discussed before, methods are tools in the service of methodological approaches. Tools in this sense are "multivocal," not wedded to a positivist or what some postmodernists would call a positivist "imperial" approach (Agger, 1998, p. 19). For example, the use of statistical procedures, such as measuring the frequency of images and texts, can reveal the saliency of a discourse and its use over time in different social contexts or media. A quantitative method is empirically grounded in the service of a postmodern approach. It is also important to point out that not all postmodernists agree with each other regarding the relative nature of the social world. As we mentioned, "postmodernism" is a term that houses a plethora of different approaches.

One defining feature of postmodern paradigms is that they assume that images, symbols, texts, and other representations have the power to create and sustain a given social reality. Thus such representations will most likely be the focus of research that proceeds from these paradigms. To illustrate postmodernist research questions that would be amenable to a mixed methods research design, we examine how a postmodernist researcher might approach what Hesse-Biber (2007) calls the "cult of thinness," a set of beliefs and practices centered around the goal of obtaining a physical ideal of slenderness.

This topic might be approached by a postmodernist researcher in terms of understanding the nature of discourses of thinness in the media. A postmodernist researcher might use a mixed methods design by conducting a qualitative content analysis of how the mainstream media constructs images of thin and overweight bodies in order to uncover messages or discourses about the ideal body. At the same time, the researcher might carry out a second, more quantitative content analysis of mainstream media images by taking a random sample of popular women's magazines over a specific period of time and counting the number of advertisements that exhibit those ideal body messages that had been uncovered in the qualitative analysis regarding the cult of thinness (Hesse-Biber, 2007). In addition, the researcher might decide to sample different types of magazines (women's vs. men's) to look for differences in discourse concerning how the cult of thinness is portrayed across magazine genres. The quantitative analysis study provides the researcher with an idea of the salience of the cult-of-thinness discourse and may even provide an opportunity to compare discourses on the cult of thinness across different print media (i.e., women's vs. men's magazines).

The questions listed in the following provide a guide to postmodernist inquiries, using this cult-of-thinness mixed methods study as an example:

- What messages or discourses are being communicated, and how?

- What are the assumptions and understandings of the female body? In our example, the researcher might ask, "How do weight loss ads in women's and men's magazines construct the 'overweight' body and the 'thin' body? What is excluded or marginalized? By whom? How?"

From a postmodernist paradigm, representations make certain definitions of reality possible while simultaneously rendering others impossible. Thus, although a photographic analysis of magazine images might reveal that thinness is associated with happiness, a postmodernist researcher might also note what is absent—that this type of photographic representation renders happiness incompatible with being "overweight." Qualitative investigation of the dominant messages about being overweight and statistical investigation of the extent or frequency of particular photograph characteristics could reveal how the photographs literally create this incompatibility.

- Are there any contradictions or inconsistencies in the text itself? Rarely is any representation or representational system completely internally coherent. On the contrary, there may be a pleth-

ora of inconsistent and confusing messages that seem to contradict one another—regarded by postmodernists as symptomatic
of a "postmodern condition." The researcher may observe that
American society pressures women to meet an ideal of thinness,
while simultaneously ridiculing them for their efforts to reach
this ideal (e.g., jokes about eating disorders).

- How do individuals and society receive the text? As we have
  stated, postmodernists contend that human society, practice,
  and identity are constituted through images, symbols, and texts.
  These both enable certain ways of being in the world and close
  off others, and postmodernists have extensively theorized about
  these allowances and limitations.

Postmodernists can *empirically* assess the effects of images, symbols,
and texts upon individuals and society. In the cult-of-thinness example,
we might follow up our qualitative findings regarding the impact of the
portrayal of women's bodies in the magazine media with a quantitative
survey of the magazines' readership concerning their own understandings and beliefs about thinness and weight loss. These quantitative data
are in the service of the postmodern perspective and are employed in
further understanding (1) the extent to which messages concerning
the thin ideal have permeated the wider society, taking on the role of a
grand narrative, and (2) the extent to which individuals who read these
magazines are in fact discerning these messages and might be affected
negatively by them. The quantitative data then act in concert with a
postmodern approach to knowledge building.

The subsequent sections contain profiles of three case studies in
which the researchers either operate entirely from a postmodern paradigm or incorporate insights from this paradigm. We use these case
studies to make *inductive* observations about mixed methods in current
postmodern research and to provide you with guidelines for engaging
in your own postmodern mixed methods study.

It is important to note that postmodernist case studies are often
difficult to profile because, first, some postmodernist and poststructuralist writers do not state that they are using a specific research method,
even those working in the social sciences. Instead, they present a theoretical discourse or social commentary with an occasional anecdote to
illustrate their point. Second, some postmodern researchers are not
always clear about the methods they use, and they may engage in a

mixed methods study without calling it that. Third and finally, it is not always easy to say whether a study is or is not postmodernist; there are often intermediate cases in which, for example, only a part of the study uses a postmodern framework or the study incorporates only limited insights from the tradition.

## Case Study 1: Researching Elite Discourse and Public Opinion in Russia

Researchers O'Loughlin, Ó Tuathail, and Kolossov (2004a, 2004b) were concerned with addressing elite discourse and public opinion in Russia. They asked the question: How do political scripts affect Russian public opinion (O'Loughlin et al., 2004a, p. 4)?

To explore this question, they conducted a content analysis of the Putin administration's discourse (i.e., speeches, writings, and editorials) regarding both the terrorist attacks of September 11, 2001, and the U.S. "war on terror" during the first 6 months after 9/11. They utilized a poststructuralist method to conduct the discourse analysis called "critical geopolitics," in which geopolitical events are deconstructed in order to reveal how they are interpretative, rather than objective, in uncovering the ways that political discourse is shaped by policy elites within a particular geopolitical state culture (p. 5).[1] Their qualitative deconstructive analysis of these data revealed that the Putin administration used a discourse that equated Russia's war against Chechen terrorists with the U.S. attacks on the Taliban and al-Qaeda, thus strategically placing Russia in alliance with the United States and the West as a "civilized" power fighting barbarians and terrorists.

Having discerned the basic elements of the discourse, O'Loughlin et al. (2004b) next wanted to look at its impact on the Russian public. To do this, they employed a quantitative component that consisted of a nationally representative survey of 1,800 adult Russians regarding their opinions about the 9/11 terrorist attacks and the subsequent war in Afghanistan. Employing a quantitative study provided the researchers with an assessment of the power of political discourse to influence public opinion.

Combining qualitative and quantitative methods in their research design, their postmodern research endeavor takes the shape of Figure 6.1.

Survey findings revealed that Russians generally endorsed the government's position on the events surrounding 9/11 and its alliance

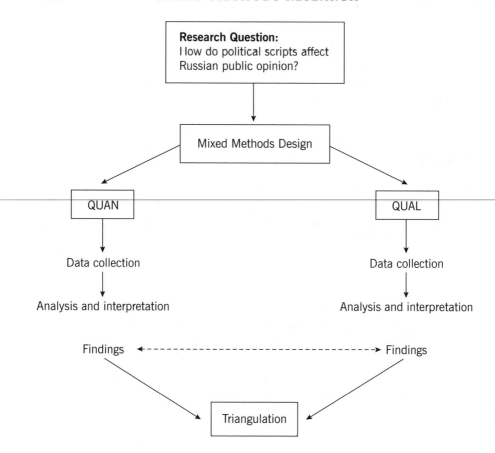

**FIGURE 6.1.** Mixed methods parallel design for Russian politics elite discourse.

with the West, though there was a smaller consensus on certain details of Putin's discourse, such as his endorsement of the West's policy of extending the war on terror to countries beyond Afghanistan.

The goal of postmodernism is to challenge dominant discourses that can hold tremendous power to shape people's perceptions and practices. The qualitative component of this study allowed the researchers to uncover the "hidden" discourse of elites that is embedded in political cultures. The quantitative component complemented the qualitative component of the study and expanded the goals of the postmodern project by discerning how dominant discourse influences public opinion. The survey revealed the extent to which dominant scripts or storylines were accepted among the larger population.

Utilizing a mixed methods design in the service of a postmodern perspective on political culture provides insights into the power of texts to construct meaning and the power that hegemonic discourse has on society. In this case, the study revealed public opinion regarding Russia's support for the United States and its response to the terrorist attacks of 9/11. Although government discourses have the power to create, shape, and sustain dominant views of geopolitical events, these findings also show that some degree of ideological autonomy may also exist among ordinary citizens, at least in Russian society.

### *Case Study 2: The Social Construction of Toxic Shock Syndrome*

In this study, Julianne Cheek (2000) drew from a postmodern perspective in order to understand how toxic shock syndrome (TSS) has been socially constructed. As a postmodernist, she was interested in the following questions:

- What different types of discourses about TSS are prevalent in the media?
- How do they influence attitudes toward those with TSS?
- What are their effects on health care praxis?

She focused her research on the Australian print media, with the goal of deconstructing the discourse with regard to their representations of TSS. For her sample, she gathered data from four Australian magazines and newspapers over a 17-year period. She employed a mixed methods analysis of print media, which involved using quantitative and qualitative methods. Her data consisted of a random sample of articles from three magazines and one newspaper, which she used in order to see the frequency, pervasiveness, and change in content of representations of TSS in the media (sampling by month, year, and type of report).

Cheek (2000) first conducted a quantitative descriptive content analysis of all these sampled articles, in which she coded for headline, topic, and visual imagery, among other categories (p. 85). This analysis provided a descriptive account that allowed her to outline "the extent, range, location, timing, and type of reporting of issues in particular media concerning Toxic Shock Syndrome" (p. 94). Second, she performed a qualitative thematic analysis that gave her a chronology of topics and themes within and across these articles. To do this, Cheek created a chronology of the sample articles, organizing them into 6-month periods.

She found that the thematic emphasis changed over the years from the issue of individual hygiene to the production of tampons. This qualitative thematic analysis of the articles allowed her to observe thematic shifts in the reporting of TSS over time.

Cheek (2000) conducted a third poststructural analysis of these data by carrying out an in-depth analysis that allowed her to uncover the hidden meanings of TSS that are portrayed in the mass media, thereby providing an opportunity to challenge dominant understandings of TSS in the public discourse. Poststructuralism (see Gannon & Davies, 2007) was originally considered a subset of postmodernism, but increasingly this term is used to focus on the power of language to shape dominant discourses within a given society. Poststructuralists contend that those in power use discourse (language) to oppress and control how others view and reproduce their reality on an ongoing basis such that it becomes "real." By deconstructing the overt and hidden meanings in dominant texts, the poststructuralist researcher reveals their power to oppress and maintain the status quo. Cheek applies a poststructural discourse analysis in which she adapts Parker's (1992) question-framing method[2] to unearth the power of the hidden meanings in her data.

Cheek (2000) identified three different discursive frameworks about TSS through her qualitative analysis: "the discourse of concealment, scientific/medical discourse and discourses about individual responsibility for health" (p. 106). The first, *discourse of concealment*, refers to an etiquette of menstruation whereby all the details of this bodily function and tampon use are treated as taboo, something to be concealed. The *scientific/medical discourse* entails hegemonic definitions of TSS as a medical problem by physicians and other scientific authorities to the exclusion of other possible definitions. Finally, *discourses of individual responsibility* define TSS as a matter of a particular woman's vigilance in taking care of herself, while relegating exterior factors (tampon production) to the margins.

Her findings revealed the power of these three qualitative frames to influence how TSS is talked about and, more important, what is not talked about, namely issues dealing with menstruation and sanitary hygiene, especially with regard to the use of sanitary products. She noted that the concealment of certain aspects of TSS protects vested economic interests (those of tampon manufacturers and health per-

sonnel who might be sued by women and their families) over those of
the people personally affected by TSS. Utilizing both quantitative and
qualitative analyses on the same dataset allowed Cheek to look at the
breadth and depth of discourse surrounding the portrayal of TSS in
print media (see Figure 6.2). In particular, the qualitative discourse
analyses enabled Cheek to get at the often hidden "competing invested
interests in how TSS is portrayed" (p. 389). Revealing the vested interests contained in TSS discourse allows less dominant groups, such as
women and their families affected by TSS, to better target their opposition to these dominant frames (p. 389). Once these alternative frames
take root in the public domain, they may then act as a catalyst for social
change in health policies and practices. This may ultimately improve

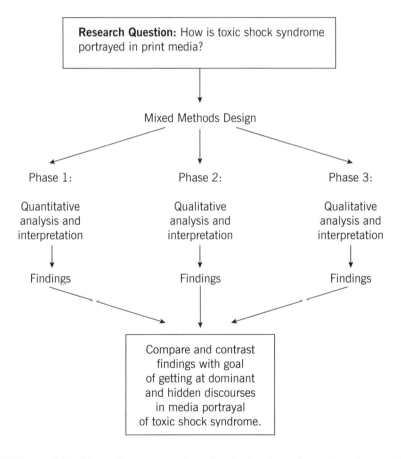

**FIGURE 6.2.** Discursive construction of toxic shock syndrome in print media.

how the media and health care providers understand medical conditions such as TSS, so that both entities can better serve the interests of those women and their families who are most affected.

### Case Study 3: Creating Social Identities on the Internet

Bowker (2001) is a postmodern researcher who used a mixed methods approach to examine the kinds of opportunities a communication technology called Internet relay chat (IRC) provides for identity exploration. A postmodern perspective views one's identity as unstable and socially malleable. Beginning with this basic assumption regarding the nature of identity allowed Bowker to explore the question of how new technologies such as the Internet provide an important landscape for experimentation with new personas and identities. Within a postmodern framework, she employed three different methods to discover how individuals construct or reconstruct identity on the Internet. She employed an exploratory parallel mixed methods design to do this.

The first component of Bowker's (2001) mixed methods study consisted of a quantitative (survey) followed by two qualitative studies, one being an ethnographic study and the other an interview study. Her explicit intention was to bring together "both positivist and interpretivist epistemologies" (2001, paragraph 29). The goal of the survey component was to determine the overall extent to which IRC participants engage in identity experimentation and exploration. For a diagram of this mixed methods design, refer to Figure 6.3.

The questions on the survey addressed the following issues, among others: whether people identified similarly both on- and offline (similar identity in terms of gender, race, etc.), whether participants' online nicknames were gender-neutral or gender-coded, the use of multiple nicknames simultaneously by one person, representing oneself as the opposite gender or a different age, and desire for a higher status position. The survey also sought demographic information in order to build a general profile of those who frequent these selected websites (paragraph 32). Bowker notes that her survey was given to 423 chat room members (316 males, 105 females) between ages 12 and 66 (2001, paragraph 31). She obtained her sample through a variety of venues that included advertising in chat rooms and newsgroups and relying on various mailing lists related to IRC.

The survey results suggested that male participants were more likely than females to experiment with their identities in IRC. Although both males and females would adopt multiple nicknames, males were more

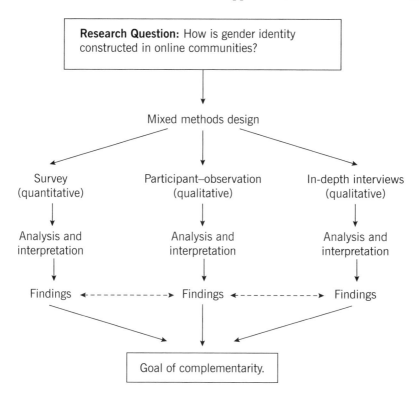

**FIGURE 6.3.** Parallel mixed methods design for identity exploration in IRC. The dashed lines represent the three methods mixing at the Findings stage.

likely to engage in "gender-switching" behavior online and to desire higher status positions online than in real life.

The qualitative component of Bowker's project was twofold. She conducted a participant–observer study of her selected online chat rooms, assuming a chat room nickname and participating in these online discussions. The ethnographic method allowed Bowker to get at the process of identity construction in real time—how IRC participants actually go about creating a self in the chat room environment. Through her analysis of online chat behaviors, she noted some important building blocks for online identities. These factors include creating a nickname, the deregulated and anarchic chat environment, and an "action command" computer function that enables participants to construct self-narratives within chat. Bowker found that, in spite of all the potential for gender identity experimentation, traditional gender roles continued to hold sway even inside the chat room.

The interview component of Bowker's qualitative study consisted of five in depth interviews with IRC participants (three males and two females). These interviews provided her with a more in-depth look at chat room participants' motivations for experimentation in the construction of online identities. She found that primary reasons for engaging in identity experimentation included protection against sexual harassment (i.e., females adopting a male identity), amusement, and testing various identity boundaries. At the same time, however, her participants also emphasized the importance of having an online persona that was stable and consistent with their real-life identities. As Bowker noted, "while it may be acceptable to adopt an alternate identity for a brief period, constant discontinuity between one's virtual and corporeal identity may be considered less permissible" (2001, paragraph 67).

Bowker's (2001) use of a mixed methods parallel exploratory design enabled her to use multiple lenses through which to view the phenomenon of identity experimentation in IRC. The survey provided a descriptive context for IRC participants' behavior, and the qualitative methods shed light on the processes and motivations involved in identity formation on the Internet. The qualitative methods also enabled her to capture the details and flux of identity formation in an everyday context. Furthermore, Bowker's mixed methods approach, rather than providing a strategy for "cross validation of theory, pursues the goal of *complementarity*, that is, convergence, by providing a fuller understanding of the research problem" (Hesse-Biber & Leavy, 2006e, p. 319). One method produced information that was absent or lacking in the others; using mixed methods allowed a more complete understanding of the phenomenon. The quantitative methods provided basic objective information about who was doing what and which factors were associated with particular types of behavior. Although a survey is limited to the questions that the researcher poses, qualitative methods enable the researcher to collect information that he or she may not have already considered. Bowker's ethnography and interviews contributed to this goal by providing further information about the details of IRC participant behavior, which gave her a broader view of the phenomenon.

This study illustrates that it is not only possible to use mixed methods from a postmodern perspective but also advantageous to do so. Because postmodern research tends to require a belief in multiple realities and varied perspectives on reality, mixed methods can be useful for providing several views of a phenomenon and for uncovering different realities. Also, the study illuminates an important reason that a postmodernist researcher might be motivated to mix methods; although positivist and postpositivist researchers assume that there is a single, knowable reality, postmodernists (as well as feminist and interpretivist researchers) tend to treat reality as multiple, complex, and incompletely knowable.

## The Benefits of a Mixed Methods Design in Postmodern Research

Postmodernism has been plagued by charges that its approach to reality is too esoteric to put into practice. Some have claimed that postmodernists are more concerned with theorizing about the nature of the social world than with actually addressing the realities of social life and creating social change (Cheek, 1999). In addition, much diversity of thought is contained under this umbrella term, such that the term itself is "highly contestable" (Bertens, 1995, p. 12). Bertens (1995) further noted that "postmodernism has been a particularly unstable concept. A single definition of postmodernism has not gone uncontested or has even been widely accepted" (as cited in Cheek, 1999, p. 384). Yet there are a set of discernable ideas within the myriad meanings of this term. Cheek (1999) encourages us to look for the similarities among the diversity of meanings. What you will find is a firm commitment to challenging modern ideas regarding knowledge building. Cheek noted that "all approaches considered to be postmodern question the assumptions embedded within modernist thought. Indeed, postmodern thought has been described as a 'crisis of confidence in the narratives of truth, science and progress that epitomized modernity'" (1999, p. 384).

A postmodernist approach to research offers a unique set of questions that challenge positivism's practice of seeking grand narratives of understanding of the social world that can obscure diversity and silence marginalized perspectives. The postmodern approach seeks to uncover a plurality of knowledges. One way it seeks to do this is through interrogating the power of discourse to create knowledge, especially those hegemonic discourses that serve to construct "universal truths." It is the task of postmodern research to question these discourses of universal truth in order to reveal the multiple layers of social life, the limitations attached to any given view of reality, and the operation of power in discourse. A postmodern mixed methods approach is particularly effective in answering questions such as:

■ What are the normative assumptions and understandings of reality?

■ Whose assumptions are these?

■ Who is included, excluded, or marginalized by this view of reality? (adapted from Cheek, 1999, p. 385)

Although the question of mixed methods in postmodernist research has not been explored previously, the three studies profiled in the previous section offer several insights into the benefits of using a mixed methods design to advance the goals of a postmodernist research agenda. Some of these benefits are outlined as follows, and some of these advantages may also pertain to other methods in the qualitative tradition:

■ *Discerning prevalence and patterning of types of discourse.* Quantitative methods can be used to determine the range and extent of specific textual features within a text, set of texts, or discourse. In the second case study, Cheek (2000) used descriptive statistics in order to determine which features—such as topics or intended audiences—are more or less prominent within her overall corpus of texts and within particular subsets (i.e., by year). Researchers are able to provide a more robust understanding of the salience of various themes and their patterning over time by combining statistics about textual characteristics with qualitative analysis of those features.

■ *Effects of discourses.* O'Loughlin and colleagues (2004a, 2004b) were able to use both types of methods—in this case, a qualitative discourse analysis and quantitative survey—to raise and ask larger questions about Russian political discourse and its impact on ordinary citizens. The qualitative component reveals the existence of certain discourses within Russian society, whereas the quantitative component investigates the extent to which Russia's citizens accept certain discourses. Because postmodernism concerns itself so extensively with how subjects and societies are constructed through images, symbols, and text, mixed methods would allow researchers to explore this insight with empirical data.

■ *Interrogating diverse perspectives.* Finally, because postmodernism emphasizes the importance of recognizing the multiplicity of perspectives on any issue or phenomenon, mixed methods provide an excellent opportunity to interrogate these diverse perspectives. Bowker (2001) uses mixed methods to achieve this objective. Her quantitative survey provides information about the prevalence of certain behaviors among specific populations and in varying contexts, and the ethnography and qualitative interviews illuminate detail that the survey could not. Sometimes, the quantitative and qualitative components of a mixed methods study may contradict one another; however, a postmodernist would likely maintain both and embrace the inconsistency by using contradictions in the data to question or deconstruct dominant assumptions or to illustrate the multiplicity of perspectives about the phenomenon studied. Table 6.1 provides an overview of the types of research questions that are amenable to mixed methods research from a postmodern perspective, based on the case studies presented in this chapter.

These are just a few of the benefits that a mixed methods design can provide to advance the agenda of postmodernist research. As more postmodernist researchers choose to incorporate quantitative methods into their work, they will likely find more uses than those mentioned here.

In the next chapter, we take you through the "nuts and bolts" of putting together a specific mixed methods research project from a qualitative approach that incorporates the advice and lessons we covered in Chapters 1–6.

**TABLE 6.1.** Types of Research Questions Amenable to a Postmodern Mixed Methods Research Design

| Question | Meaning | Studies |
|---|---|---|
| What are the effects of discourses and their impact on the target population? | Interplay between hegemonic texts and discourses and everyday society | O'Loughlin, Ó Tuathail, & Kolossov (2004a, 2004b) |
| What textual features are most prevalent in media discourse and how do these representations change over time? | Range and extent and change in textual and discursive features within a particular text, text set, or discourse | Cheek (2000) |
| How is identity constructed on the Internet in relation to one's traditional gendered role? | Effects of discourses and texts on possibilities of information and knowledge | Bowker (2001) |

## GLOSSARY

**affirmative postmodernism:** accepts that some versions of reality are truer than others but rejects the idea of one "truth."

**critical geopolitics:** in this framework, geopolitical events are considered interpretative, shaped by elite policymakers in a particular state or culture. It sees geopolitics (the study of geography, history, and social sciences) as a set of discourses and practices rather than an objective science.

**deconstruction:** a critique that aims to analyze the information that is left out of a text, the "other" that is the opposite of what the text affirms.

**discourses:** broad term that includes images, symbols, and texts or any form of visual or other communication.

**metanarrative:** (also grand narrative) any conceptual system that purports to subsume all of reality within its own universe of meaning, for example, Christianity and Marxism.

**postcolonialism:** intellectual theories developed as a reaction to political colonialism that deal with cultural identity in colonized and formerly colonized societies.

**postmodernism:** viewpoint that challenges the status quo of modern enlightenment thought, rejects the idea of universal truths, and accepts subjectivity and multiple legitimate interpretations.

**poststructuralism:** intellectual movement that rejects the concept of objective "truths," holds that there is no singular "self" identity, and replaces authors with readers as the primary creators of meaning.

**queer theory:** field of thought that seeks to understand all forms of sexual behavior and identity, built on feminist and gay/lesbian studies.

**skeptical postmodernism:** sees all interpretations of reality as equally valid, making the idea of accurately describing social reality impossible and irrelevant. Rejects the idea of "theory," because no theory can be more correct than another.

### DISCUSSION QUESTIONS

1. In what way(s) does a postmodern perspective lend itself to analyzing multicultural perspectives and narratives within sociology? What sets postmodern perspectives apart from other commonly accepted, more dominant approaches?

**2.** With regard to issues such as eating disorders, how might postmodernism be implemented to better analyze these social phenomena?

**3.** Does questioning universal truth really lead to unbiased research? Can postmodernism still be effective despite repudiating commonly accepted research approaches like positivism?

■ ■ ■ SUGGESTED WEBSITES ■ ■ ■

### Postmodernism

*www.edu.plymouth.ac.uk/resined/postmodernism/pmhome.htm*

This site provides detailed background on postmodernism and specifically discusses postmodern education research with case studies.

### NOTES

1. As Hesse-Biber and Leavy (2006e) noted:

> Deconstruction . . . is a method of conducting an internal critique of texts. In essence, a deconstructive approach to textual analysis aims at exposing what is concealed with what has been left out of a text. . . . It is based on the notion that the meaning of words happens in relation to sameness and difference. In every text, some things are affirmed, such as truth, meaning, and authorship/authority; however, there is always an "other" that contrasts with that which is affirmed. This other . . . appears absent from the text but is actually contained within the text as different or deferred. . . . The aim of deconstruction . . . [is] to displace assumptions within the text . . . this process shows that the meaning of a text is never single or fixed. (pp. 292–293)

2. These framing questions (Parker, 1992) are geared toward extracting both dominant and hidden discourses in the data. The framing questions that Cheek employed for each article were:

   ■ What did the study uncover?

   ■ What discursive frames influenced the way TSS was represented in the media?

   ■ What was the effect of these frames?

   ■ What implications do the findings of this study have for health care practice?

# CHAPTER 7

# Putting It Together

## Qualitative Approaches
## to Mixed Methods Research Praxis

This chapter provides a hands-on experience in conducting a mixed methods project using a qualitative approach. We walk through an in-depth case study by providing a step-by-step commentary on how to put the variety of skills and knowledge we have gained into mixed methods research practice. The praxis of mixed methods will take a back-and-forth approach that includes tapping into our creative energy and newly acquired knowledge of the range of analytical and interpretative mixed methods skills. We may find moments of great discovery and generation of theoretical insights into the analysis and interpretation of this case study. We may also find ourselves developing a tolerance for some chaos and ambiguity. It is a journey well worth taking, for it ultimately creates and grows our potential for acquiring a more complex understanding of the social world.

In this chapter, I provide a research example that illustrates the genesis and analysis of a qualitative mixed methods research project. This study has *not* actually been conducted. I created this research project in order to illustrate the range of mixed methods practices discussed in this book. The interview material I present, however, is from an actual interview I conducted with a male ex-football player who is now a trainer. All the research literature cited comes from studies on the topic of body image, and I have listed several other research examples that tackle this type of problem, though not from a mixed methods vantage point. Although I cannot tackle all the qualitative approaches talked about, I selected a general qualitative interpretative approach to mixed methods, and together we follow this approach from the inception of the research question or set of questions to the selection of a research design and then proceed to the analysis and writing up stages of the project. I provide a general set of critical questions, guidelines, and checklists along the way that bring together many of the issues discussed in Chapters 1–6. These tips are presented in the form of sections titled "Research Praxis Aside." All research praxis asides are shaded to differentiate them from our ongoing research example. These asides are not inclusive of all the things you might need to ask in your own particular study, but they are general enough to be applicable to many qualitative approaches to mixed methods. It is important to consider adding or deleting certain questions in order to model these research praxis ideas for your own use. The research praxis section can be envisioned as a series of reflexive moments in which the researcher engages throughout the research process. Although this specifically applies to mixed methods research from a qualitative approach, many of these questions also apply to any type of research project, whether from a qualitative or quantitative set of approaches.

## Putting It into Practice: Conducting a Qualitative Approach to a Mixed Methods Research Project

### Setting the Scene: A Qualitative Mixed Methods Research Project Example

Men today have rigorous standards when it comes to their bodies. The ideal, attractive male has defined muscles from his shoulders, arms, and chest to his abs, legs, and calves. He has a structured jaw line and a full head of hair but a chest without any hair. Men in the media are young and toned, recruited to sell items from paper towels to diet soda. Men struggling to express their masculinity are increasingly concerned about their body image and are spending hours in the gym, lifting weights and trying to bulk up. I spoke with a trainer named Mike at my local gym in Boston, Massachusetts, about the issue of men and body image. This is Mike's response to a question concerning whom the men at this gym compare themselves with:

"I think more each other. You know? I think it should be more of a self impression than it is anything else and no matter how much an individual looks at each other or themselves in general it's never good enough. They are never either big enough, they are never either cut enough so they'll go to any extreme, to all extremes to get to their goals."

When asked to give his thoughts on why the men were so overly concerned with their bodies, he replied:

"Attraction, I think, and that's the main, main issue; sexual attraction to the opposite sex. It could be figuring to match up with individuals if you're looking at it at a manly base, or it's an ego thing . . . it's how you look at yourself compared to other people."

Later in the interview, Mike spoke about his own sense of esteem and body image, and how he felt about men using steroids:

"It's like I always had to be the best. So I would always train. I mean I used to get, like even in high school, I'd go to the gym in the morning, you know to work out. I'd go to school, I have practice, I'd go to the gym afterwards. I was probably one of the very few, only kids in high school that did that. . . . "

"Um, off season I was the only one that actually started to, you know, train directly off season. I had [football] coaches that would help me. . . . I had a friend of the family, uh, that would . . . come down from, um, he was a football star for a large Big Ten school and he worked one on one with an Olympics training coach, so he came down to help me out a lot."

Mike revealed to me that he in fact has used supplements to enhance his already muscular look:

"I'm not going to say I've never taken ephedrine [a chemical stimulant used as an energy booster and to improve athletic performance], I do now. I've taken it because I see the results. I'm not the type of person that says I need more, because I know more is better. I don't take more than I need. I'll take the serving or half a serving, you know? It's only a little thing again, it speeds your metabolism up just a little bit more energy, where it makes you sweat a little bit even more. You know it gives you a little bit more energy per set. So it's more of a charge, like having a coffee in the morning, to wake you up, it's the same concept."

Despite having used performance-enhancing drugs, Mike personally knows the risks of using steroids to obtain more muscle:

"One individual actually used to be a friend of my friend's, I wasn't a real good friend of him but I was associated with him, just passed away. He was 23 years old. He gained 110 pounds of solid muscle, in one year. That's almost impossible. And not understanding that, that his heart is also a muscle that also built and built and built to a point where it just burst in his sleep. . . . For men, wanting to look good is asking 'Am I big enough?' . . . where people try to, think that they have to be diced. Meaning very defined, very muscular, um, in comparing themselves to everybody else."

### A Short Literature Review Introducing the Research Problem

In their new book, *The Adonis Complex: The Secret Crisis of Male Body Obsession,* Harrison Pope, Katharine Phillips, and Roberto Olivardi (2000) noted that within the past two decades, men have become obsessed with having a "well built and muscular" body image (p. 30). Men desire enhanced muscle definition as part of their ideal body. Pope and his colleagues researched more than 1,000 males over a 15-year period and suggested that men desire to look like Adonis, "half man and half god— the ultimate in masculine beauty" (p. 6). Increasingly, steroid use has been an integral part of producing men's "bulkier" look. They noted that men desire to look big and muscular in large part to offset what they see as women's increasing power within society. Eating disorders are rising in record numbers among the male population, and, in fact, a new disorder they labeled "bigorexia" has developed among young males (p. 11). This disorder causes men who are muscular to be unable to judge their own body image (body dysmorphia). They look in a mirror and feel that their bodies are frail and that they need to further increase their muscle size by taking steroids and excessively lifting weights.

### Male Body Dissatisfaction

The emphasis on male body "perfection" appears to be becoming ever more invasive as there is growing evidence that men are becoming increasingly dissatisfied with their weight and body image. In 1992, Gustafson Larson and Terry compared body dissatisfaction between adolescent girls and boys. Although their research showed higher rates of body disturbance among the female population, a shocking 45% of the boys wanted to change their weight as well—38% wanted to be thinner. This stunning finding spawned additional research that supports the contention that male body image dissatisfaction is a serious concern that must be studied. Cohane and Pope (2001) conducted a literature review of studies regarding body image and boys that concluded that there had been a "striking increase in body image concerns among men" (p. 373). They also concluded that, similarly to girls, body image closely correlates with self-esteem in boys. The high numbers of boys who are dissatisfied with their bodies, whether they feel too small or too big, is thus an important category for further sociological inquiry.

Additional research also concludes that as men are becoming increasingly dissatisfied with their bodies, they are increasingly connecting their self-esteem to their body image ("Pumping Up Your Body Image," 2002; "Body Image: Equal Opportunity Anxiety," 2002). A recent study of body dissatisfaction in men noted that 25% of men surveyed in 1972 were dissatisfied with their bodies and that that number increased to 67% by 1997 ("Pumping Up," 2002). All of this research advocates for the need for further in-depth research on why this increase in body dissatisfaction is occurring in male populations, what the specific issues are, and how men are handling it.

### RESEARCH PRAXIS ASIDE 1. ASSESSING THE "BIG PICTURE"

In order to begin our research journey, let's lay out the steps one would need to address along the way, and then we can tackle each one as we go along.

• *Step 1.* Determine what you want to study and develop a finely tuned research problem. Qualitative research problems usually focus on understanding the subjective experience as a source of knowledge building. Although you will not necessarily be testing out specific hypotheses that are stated up front, you will need to create a focused research question.

Reviewing the research literature is often an important first step toward helping you to formulate and/or fine-tune your research question. The literature review does not have to be extensive in the beginning of your project. It is likely that your research question will shift once you begin to analyze and interpret the first round of data collected. Insights from this early data may, in fact, find you shifting the questions you ask, and you may find yourself consulting a new research literature and so on (you might go back to Chapter 2 for tips on putting together your literature review).

Given your initial research question, it is important to determine whether or not a mixed methods study design is appropriate for this research problem. To do so, jot down in one paragraph your research justification for using mixed methods. In writing this paragraph, be sure to think about the link between the problem and the method (to remind yourself of this process, refer back to Chapter 2).

• *Step 2*. Determine what type of mixed methods design would be appropriate for this type of research problem (refer back to Chapter 3). It might be useful to ask yourself whether your research design is iterative in nature. You may have a specific design in mind, but you should be open to a range of designs as your research project proceeds. Don't close off opportunities for reconfiguring your design in response to research results.

• *Step 3*. Determine how you will approach your data collection. What type of data do you intend to collect and why? This will depend on the mixed methods design you selected in Step 2 (refer to Chapter 3 here, especially the section on sampling and data collection).

• *Step 4*. Determine what type of analysis you will conduct on your collected data. Will you integrate your analysis and interpretation from each study or will you conduct separate analyses? At what stage will you integrate these data, if at all?

• *Step 5*. How will you write up your study? Will you write up each study separately? Will you integrate findings from all studies in your write up? Please refer back to Chapter 3 for more guidelines.

### Mixed Methods Research Example: The Lived Experience of College Football Players

We start out with a research example derived from some ideas that came out of my interview with an ex-college football player, as well as a short literature review performed around the same subject area. Although the general goal of our study is to understand lived experiences of college football players (both during their playing time and afterward), we are also particularly interested in finding out their feelings about their body image and self-esteem, as well as any exposure to and/or firsthand experience with enhancement drug use during their college sports careers. We break our study down into the steps previously outlined.

## Step 1. Research Problem Stage:
### The Mixed Methods Research Problem

For our example, the research problem includes the following questions:

- What is the lived experience of a male college football player?

- How do male college football players feel about their bodies?

- To what extent, if any, is the use of performance-enhancement drugs part of their experience as athletes?

- How prevalent is the use of performance-enhancement drugs and/or supplements among college football players? To what extent, if any, do they perceive it to be part of the lived experience of other college football players in general?

---

### RESEARCH PRAXIS ASIDE 2. THE RESEARCH PROBLEM

Most researchers embarking on a new mixed methods research project must grapple with the following question:

- How do I come up with a research problem?

The following are a set of sensitizing questions that might help you start out as you seek a workable research problem on this issue or, for that matter, any research problem you may be struggling with.

- What is my researcher standpoint?

- Are there other stakeholders involved in this research problem genesis?

- Do I have the skills to complete this project? If not, should I consider a team-based approach?

- To what extent will I need to incorporate different methodological (theoretical) approaches and methods to this issue? How will I integrate these different methodological perspectives and methods, if at all, throughout the research process?

- Do I have the resources to complete this study?

- Do I have the time to accurately and faithfully complete this study?

- How will a review of the research literature on this topic assist me with the formulation of my research problem? Will the literature review be conducted at the beginning, or will it be iterative and referred back to throughout the research process?

## Step 2. Determining Your Mixed Methods Research Design

This study uses a *mixed methods sequential explanatory approach,* as illustrated in Figure 7.1.

The first study (hereby referred to as Phase 1) consists of an anonymous semistructured Internet survey of a convenience sample of former football players who were listed at any time in their college football careers as "starting string" players in "Big Ten" football and who have either graduated or left their universities within the past 5 years. The purpose of this survey was to ascertain the prevalence of performance-enhancement drugs among football players, as well as to understand whether there were any differences in use by race, socioeconomic status, and ethnicity. The survey consisted of 40 survey questions that covered basic demographic information, as well as a set of scales from our literature review that measured psychological and social factors associated with the usage of enhancement drugs. The survey also included assessment of the frequency and extent of this usage during their college athletic careers and their knowledge about how widespread enhancement drug use was among their fellow teammates.

The purpose of Phase 1 of this study was to gather an overall context within which we could assess the use of enhancement drugs in the college football environment, as well as to assist with the gathering of a subsample of respondents for a qualitative study of their lived

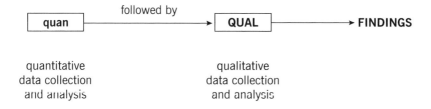

**FIGURE 7.1.** Mixed methods sequential explanatory design.

experience as college athletes. Phase 1 of the study also provided some key questions that we might expand on in our in-depth interview. We especially wanted to use the survey results from Phase 1 to gauge the representativeness of our Phase 2 subpopulation, and also utilize the information to generalize and/or extend the findings we gathered from Phase 2 by comparing and contrasting the results of some of our findings from Phase 1 and 2 on those questions that appeared to cover the same material.

## RESEARCH PRAXIS ASIDE 3.
## SELECTION OF A MIXED METHODS DESIGN

Once you have asked yourself the guiding questions from Step 1, you will have a question or set of questions to answer in the research project. Next, we focus on important guidelines to consider when deciding what mixed methods design best suits your project:

- What is the link between the research problem and the research method?

- In what sense does this research problem lend itself to this type of methods design?

- Am I open and flexible to design change?

- What will be my primary and secondary methods?

- Will I use qualitative methods followed by quantitative, quantitative followed by qualitative, or perhaps two qualitative studies?

- In what temporal manner will I implement them? In other words, will one method come first, or will they be performed sequentially? Or will it be a parallel study?

- At what stage(s) in the research process will I mix methods?

### Step 3. Data Collection Stage

Sampling techniques for Phase 1 were eclectic, ranging from snowball sampling to perusing the football archives of Big Ten universities in order to locate names of past starting players. In order to locate the list of players, I also used the Internet and perused various websites, including Facebook and MySpace. Additionally, I solicited respondents through postings about the study on a range of football websites, where

I obtained permission to post a query asking users who met the sample criteria to contact me if they were interested in participating in the study. The final sample consisted of 400 semistructured questionnaires on which the analysis of Phase 1 was based. All interviews were anonymous and were administered over the Internet.

At the end of the interview, in a separate section of the survey not linked to their responses, respondents had the option of checking off whether they were interested in participating in a follow-up phone interview. I also asked those who were interested in being contacted for an in-depth interview whether or not they would agree to have their surveys linked to their subsequent interviews.

I sent all those who expressed an interest more information about the phone interview, along with a consent form that they electronically signed and sent back to me with times that they were available for a phone interview.

Phase 2 consisted of a subsample of 100 ex-football players gathered from Phase 1, who agreed to an in-depth telephone interview concerning their lived experience as college football players. Out of these 100 interviews, 40 respondents also agreed to the matching up of their in-depth interviews with their previous survey questionnaires.

During this period, I needed to obtain approval to conduct this study from my college's institutional review board (IRB) by following a specific university protocol. To do this, I needed to write up a short proposal that followed the IRB guidelines and to develop a set of semistructured questions for Phase 1 that dealt with assessing body image satisfaction, the extent and frequency of performance-enhancement drug use, the frequency and type of exercise regimen practiced while playing football, and so on. I submitted these questions to the IRB, along with a set of open-ended questions I planned to ask respondents in Phase 2 and a detailed consent form for their approval. Respondents had to agree to and sign a consent form before the interview process began. For an example of mixed methods consent forms, please see Appendix 7.1.

## RESEARCH PRAXIS ASIDE 4. ETHICAL ISSUES IN MIXED METHODS RESEARCH

Meeting the requirements of an IRB and conducting ethical research should be a foremost concern of all mixed methods researchers. Consider the following guidelines as you think about the potential ethical complications and pitfalls of your project, as well as how you will collect a sample for your study:

- What ethical issues can I potentially foresee from my research question and research design?

- Have I ethically obtained my research sample? What rules or guidelines apply to conducting sampling using the Internet or other technologies in which I do not have face-to-face contact with the research participant?

- What responsibility do I have toward my research participant? For example, do I have their informed consent to participate in my project?

- What ethical issues/dilemmas might come into play in deciding what research findings I publish?

- Will my research directly benefit those who participated in the study?

- What will I do to ensure the privacy of my respondents? What kind of confidentiality agreement can I offer those who participate in my research project?

- What ethical framework and philosophy informs my work and ensures respect and sensitivity for those I study, beyond whatever may be required by law?

## Sampling Concerns in Mixed Methods Research

Mixed methods sampling designs should flow from one's underlying research problem or set of problems. A qualitatively driven research approach may employ a concurrent sampling design (QUAN + QUAL) with the goal of improving the validity of the qualitative research findings. A qualitatively driven researcher may use a sequential sampling design to test out ideas generated from a qualitative study by collecting data on a representative population (QUAL → quan). A sequential design employing a quantitative study first is often used when the researcher seeks to gain perspective on what results seem important and worthy of further in-depth exploration (quan → QUAL). In addition, a qualitatively driven researcher might employ a sequential design in order to increase the validity of his or her qualitative findings by using the quantitative sample to inform the specific type of subsequent qualitative sample chosen. For example, the findings from a quantitative sample can provide the criteria for determining the particular population selected for a qualitative sample.

## RESEARCH PRAXIS ASIDE 5. SAMPLING ISSUES IN MIXED METHODS RESEARCH: FINDING A DELICATE BALANCE

One of the most important issues to consider when sampling in a mixed methods project is how to connect your sampling decisions to your research question.

In thinking about the *quantitative method phase* of your mixed methods study with regard to sample issues, you might ask:

- What is my target population or set of populations for this phase?

- Will I be using the quantitative method to provide me with a representative sample of the target population as defined by my study? If so, I will need to make sure that I have been careful to conduct a random sample from which I can ultimately generalize my research results. I will need to decide on the specific type of random sample depending on my research question.

- Have I made sure the sample size is adequate to answer my research question?

- Have I carefully determined that my sampling frame is, in fact, representative of the target population under study?

In thinking about the *qualitative phase* of this project and sampling issues, you might ask the following:

- What is my target population?

- Does the sample I collect need to be representative of the wider target population? If so, how can I obtain a representative qualitative sample?

- Will I rely on data I collect from my quantitative study to directly link to my qualitative study to inform my sample?

- Should I nest my qualitative study in the quantitative one and collect in-depth data from all respondents at the same time? Why or why not?

- Is the qualitative sample size adequate to answer the research question?

*For both samples ask:*

- Do the sampling designs follow ethical guidelines set forth by such entities as the IRB?

*Turning a Research Topic into a Quantitative Approach
to a Mixed Methods Project*

Before moving on to the analysis and interpretation section of our mixed methods project, let's address how we could have turned this general research topic into a quantitative approach to a research project instead of the qualitative approach we have used.

We would first need to reframe the research problem, perhaps starting out with the following set of questions:

- What social and psychological factors best predict performance-enhancement drug usage among student athletes? Do these factors differ by the race or ethnic background of the athlete?

- Do the key factors found in this study triangulate with the lived experiences of a small subsample of college athletes?

These research questions would probably come from an intense literature review, looking to specifically identify a prior set of specific variables that have been shown to predict high levels of enhancement drug use among athletes. We might also come up with a range of hypotheses that deal with differences among athletes in terms of race and ethnicity. Some literature, for example, suggests that rates of different types of drug use are higher among European American student athletes (see Green, Uryasz, Petr, & Bray, 2001).

To begin a literature review, you might peruse a variety of social science databases available online and begin searching, using key words such as "social factors," "psychological factors," "social psychological factors," "performance-enhancing drugs," "college athletes," and "athletes," looking for empirical studies on this topic. In fact, when I perused the literature, I came up with a variety of articles, including an excellent review of this literature (see Kirby, Moran, Guerin, & MacIntyre, 2008).

Given our quantitative approach to the research problem in this example, we might decide on a sequential explanatory design (quantitative data collection followed by qualitative data collection). To see an example, refer to Figure 7.2.

In this type of model, the researcher prioritizes the quantitative data and analysis and collects these data first. The qualitative study (Phase 2) is used very often in the service of the quantitative study (Phase 1) to "follow up" on some issues or results that the researcher seeks to understand more in depth, perhaps refining some particular quanti-

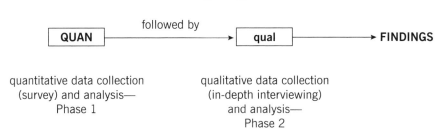

**FIGURE 7.2.** Mixed methods sequential explanatory design: A possible quantitative approach.

tative measures for a subsequent survey (for an example of conducting a quantitative mixed methods model on the topic of performance-enhancement drug use, see Kirby et al., 2008). More important, in this study the researcher seeks to validate the quantitative study by checking the results against an in-depth sample of ex-college football players, looking for the extent to which the findings from one study (Phase 1) are corroborated by the findings from the other study (Phase 2).

We might also conduct a quantitative mixed methods study by asking yet another set of questions. For example, suppose it were the case that we knew very little about drug use among athletes in general and football players in particular. Suppose reading the literature showed that few studies on this topic had been done. Instead of launching into a larger survey research project whose goal was to test out hypotheses about the correlates of drug use among college athletes, we might start with a smaller in-depth qualitative study whose goal was to identify questions for our survey that were grounded in an understanding of the everyday experiences of athletes. Our ultimate goal would be to test out some specific hypotheses on drug use, as well as to assess the prevalence of drug use. To carry out our new project goals, we would begin by conducting an exploratory mixed methods sequential study, as follows (see Figure 7.3).

In this type of project, we would first conduct a qualitative in-depth study whose purpose would be to identify particular themes from the respondents' own experiences, looking in particular for any associations between specific motivations for using enhancement drugs and the respondent's roles as athletes. We might even want to separate out our in-depth findings into those from respondents who had high drug use and those from respondents who had low drug use while involved in college athletics. From these data, we could try to generate a set of hypotheses that we could explore using a larger quantitative survey of

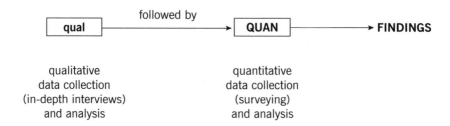

**FIGURE 7.3.** Mixed methods sequential exploratory design: Another possibility.

ex-college football players. The qualitative study would then serve as an exploratory study whose purpose is to generate hypotheses and to explore any relationships we may find in these data for further testing.

It is important for one to look at the researcher's rationale for conducting a mixed methods study and to question the researcher's use of a particular mixed methods design. You will notice in comparing the various designs that we have employed on this topic that the first mixed methods designs we discussed in this praxis chapter (see Figure 7.1) looks quite similar to the mixed methods designs of the qualitative approach presented earlier and that both mixed methods designs begin with a quantitative study followed by a qualitative study (see Figure 7.2). Both mixed methods models are sequential designs. What makes them different is the emphasis placed on the quantitative and qualitative portions. In addition, one must also look into the motivation underlying any mixed methods design. The first study (the one we are following through) aims to explore and understand the lived experiences of college athletes, whereas the second study is positioned to explain the underlying set of causal factors that lead to performance-enhancement drug use. Each design has a different set of underlying motivations that emanate from the specific set of research problems each study seeks to address.

### Step 3, Continued.
### Specific Data Collection Techniques

#### Phase 1: Survey Research Project

Having identified the target population and the type of survey to employ, I created a series of survey questions that were pretested on a small population of ex-football players. I also included a performance-enhancement drug use attitude inventory that had a high degree of validity and reliability. I chose an online e-mail survey to administer the questionnaire (for more specifics on how to conduct an online survey and their strengths and weaknesses, see Andrews, Nonnecke, & Preece, 2003).

## Phase 2: In-Depth Interview Project

I conducted 100 phone interviews using an open-ended interview with some semistructured questions based on information I thought was important from Phase 1. Let's take a look at how I, as a white, middle-class, female college professor, conducted these interviews, keeping in mind that each of us, as researchers, bring our own particular life experiences to the interview process (and to keep this in mind, we practice reflexivity, as mentioned in Chapter 3). I started out the interview with a set of general, open-ended interview questions with the goal of gaining insight and understanding into the respondents' lives during the time they played football in college. At this time, I am mindful that I am an "outsider"—a white, middle-class, female college professor who is interviewing male ex-football players. In my interviews, I must remain conscious and question how I will negotiate the range of differences that go beyond issues of gender (e.g., other differences in terms of my race/ethnicity and possibly class status). It would be important at this point for me to reflect in a research memo on these differences and how they might influence the research situation; as researchers, all our memos would be individual and bring up different issues of divergence and convergence, depending on our viewpoints. A few good themes or questions to consider in such a memo include the following:

- How do my unique differences conflict with those I interview?

- How do these differences affect the perception and responsiveness of the ex-athlete I am interviewing?

- What biases do I bring to the interview situation?

Reflexivity is key at all points in the research process, especially, in this example, at the beginning of data collection.

We can gather our data by using a digital recorder hooked up to the telephone. We should be careful at the end of each interview to ask each respondent if there is something he (or she) would like to talk about that we have not touched on. We also remain aware of the valuable data that can emerge when we officially end the interview but continue to talk with our respondent. We should be careful to consider what we have learned about the importance of establishing rapport with our respondents and of listening intently to what they are telling us, mindful of any muted language contained within their dialogue.

### Step 4. Data Analysis and Interpretation

Once we begin to collect research data, it is time to begin to analyze our findings and fit the pieces of the research puzzle together. We do not gather all the interview data at once, doing one interview right after the other. Instead, after each interview we conduct for a research project, we immerse ourselves in the data we have collected by playing back the recording. As we begin to transcribe the interview, we also begin to analyze and interpret our data. That is, we write down any ideas that come to mind ("memoing") and note the themes that we find particularly important. After a few interviews, we should especially look for the common pathways or patterns of behavior by which individuals experience their bodies within a college football culture. We would be particularly mindful to write down our ideas as a set of data memos.

---

**RESEARCH PRAXIS ASIDE 6.**
**ANALYSIS AND INTERPRETATION GUIDELINES**

When beginning to collect data and think about how you will use them in analysis and interpretation, consider the following questions:

- How will I perform my data analysis? Will I integrate software such as CAQDAS into my analysis and interpretation?

- Have the findings of both methods been thoroughly addressed and integrated (if possible)? Have I privileged one method over the other?

- At what points do my findings agree or disagree with each other?

- Have I practiced reflexivity throughout my data collection and analysis?

---

*Coding an Interview*

The key to data analysis is to search for meanings within the data. *Memoing* and *coding* are two important ways to do so. In the following segment of text, we can see an excerpt from interviews with Mike, ex-collegiate football player and current trainer, concerning his feelings about his body.

| Interview Text Segment | Line-by-Line Coding |
|---|---|
| "I'm not going to say I've never taken ephedrine, I do now. I've taken it because I see the results. I'm not the type of person that says I need more, because I know more is better. I don't take more than I need. I'll take the serving or half a serving, you know? It's only a little thing again, it speeds your metabolism up just a little bit more energy, where it makes you sweat a little bit even more. You know it gives you a little bit more energy per set. So it's more of a charge, like having a coffee in the morning, to wake you up, it's the same concept." | Takes enhancement drugs<br><br>Drugs give you "results"<br>Importance of not getting addicted to drugs:<br>  Not taking "more than you need"<br>Drugs give results:<br>  Speed up metabolism<br>  Gives you energy<br><br>Normalizing drug use:<br>  More of a charge, "like having coffee" |

As you can see from this excerpt, I have coded the first few lines of text from one interview using a *literal coding procedure* that uses the respondent's own words. These are *descriptive code categories*. If we proceed down the code list, we see that the coding becomes more *analytical*; the phrase "normalizing drug use" is an excellent illustration of this shift. Nowhere does the respondent directly say this, but the researcher is able to generate the more conceptual code of "normalizing" by building from the respondent's words.

We should remember that to code means to take a segment of text and give it a "name" or sometimes a number. There are many ways to code a given text. We began by doing some literal coding and moved quickly to a more *focused coding procedure*. Sociologist Kathy Charmaz (1995) uses the term "focused coding" and suggests that the researchers look at all the data they have coded from the interview. In our example, the researchers would look at "positive body image" and consider each piece of text associated with that code for each interview. The researchers could then compare each segment with the others in order to come up with a clearly delineated working idea of what the concept "positive body image" means (Charmaz, 1983, p. 117).

Focused coding differs from literal coding in that we are not placing a "label" on something to describe what it is; rather, we are looking for a code description that allows us to develop an understanding or interpretation of what our respondents are saying about their body image. To engage in focused coding means to sort our literal codes into more abstract categories. This modification of code categories is a process that moves our analysis from a literal to a more abstract level. This method is important in order to generate theoretical ideas.

We might begin this process in earnest after coding a number of interviews with college athletes and retrieving the texts associated with specific codes. Let's refer to the previous segment of text. Suppose that we retrieved all the text associated with the code "drugs." When we read through all of the text segments associated with this code, we are able to see that respondents are, in fact, talking about the use of drugs in a variety of ways. For example, in the preceding text segment, I noted all those codes associated with drugs: "drugs give you results," "not getting addicted," "drugs give you energy." Contained within these codes are motivations for drug use, as well as justification for drug use. As I continued to memo about the meaning of how Mike thinks about the term "drug use," I began to liken his lived experiences to French philosopher and sociologist Michel Foucault's (1975) definition of "normalization," whereby Mike frames his drug use as a normal part of his everyday practice and it becomes "normal" through a process that pairs his drug use with a set of readily acceptable reasons for using (Foucault, 1975, p. 184). By repeating statements about using drugs within this justification frame—"drugs give you energy," "drugs work"—and saying he knows his limits (not becoming addicted), drug use becomes a normal part of Mike's life (for more on the concept of normalization, see Foucault, 1975).

In future interviews, we might look for other types of normalization practices concerning drug use and also perhaps look at the ways that college athletes practice "body surveillance," which is the idea that male athletes are constantly watching and monitoring their bodies. This can include checking for muscle mass, watching their images in the mirror, weighing themselves several times during the day, and comparing their bodies with those of other male athletes. With this example, we can see how the initial codes then become part of a larger conceptual category that, overall, captures the importance of surveillance as a "control mechanism" used to coax men's bodies toward the muscular ideal initiated by the self and society. We can see how we are moving our analysis from the literal plane to a more abstract and theoretical understanding of male athletes' use of drugs and its relationship to male body image concerns. We might then begin to look at differences among the sample of college athletes to determine whether race, ethnicity, and class cause differences in drug use.

Initial codes in the body image study were changed as follows:

| From: | To: |
|-------|-----|
| Drugs give you energy | Motivation for drug use |
| Drugs give you results | Motivation for drug use |
| Drugs give you a charge | Motivation for drug use |
| Not becoming addicted | Knowing your limits |
| Motivation for drug use | Normalization practices |
| Knowing your limits | Normalization practices |

In analyzing these data, we may consider employing *grounded theory*, which acts as both theory and method in that it allows researchers to analyze their findings by developing "progressively more abstract conceptual categories to synthesize, to explain and to understand" (Charmaz, 1995, p. 28). To do this, we code the text line by line, a technique Charmaz calls "open coding." As we do so, we ask ourselves several questions:

- What is going on?

- What are people doing?

- What do these actions and statements take for granted? (Charmaz, 1995, p. 38)

In this type of analysis, memoing becomes key to formulating major ideas about what is going on in the data. You should be taking memos during all steps of the research analysis stage, and it is important to return back to your memos in order to compare and elaborate on ideas that you may have had about your data but were previously unable to verify. Memoing may ultimately reveal information that you notice only on a second or third look back.

We have applied a grounded theory analysis to these data; however, there are other methods for analyzing your data. One of these might be to conduct a *narrative analysis*, in which, as opposed to the line reading used in grounded theory, the researcher looks at the data as a whole and concentrates on the types of narratives (stories) told by the participant to you as a researcher. The following questions are useful to ask in a narrative analysis:

- What structure does the story take?

- What events or episodes does the participant describe?

- What are the meanings of the stories told?

This type of analysis can be very useful, depending on which method the researcher deems most helpful in uncovering the meaning of the respondents' stories. Because research is an iterative process, we can choose several ways of analyzing (i.e., identifying what the data say) and interpreting (understanding what that means).

*The Iterative Process in the Analysis and Interpretation of Data*[1]

As Figure 7.4 illustrates, the research process is fluid; the researcher is constantly engaged in data collection, analysis, and interpretation of research findings in dynamic ways. As the researcher goes through the research process, it is important that she or he constantly examines her or his memos and looks for any new connections.

---

### RESEARCH PRAXIS ASIDE 7. REVIEWING YOUR MEMOS

The following are some questions you may want to consider as you go back and review your memo notes:

- Which of my memo ideas are supported by the data? Are any not supported?

- What do my memos tell me about my research question and the data I have collected?

- Are there questions I haven't asked but should?

- Do I need to extend my sample or interview questions?

- Are there outliers or data I have not addressed?

- Have I followed up on all data I could follow up on?

---

Sociologist David Karp, with whom we have become familiar "behind the scenes" in previous chapters, offers the following observation on early memoing:

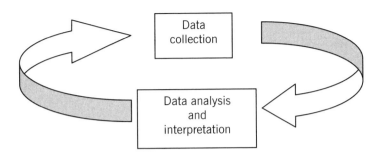

**FIGURE 7.4.** Iterative approach to data analysis. Adapted from Hesse-Biber and Leavy (2006a). Copyright 2006 by Sage Publications, Inc. Adapted by permission.

*Especially at the beginning, you will hear people say things that you just hadn't thought about. Look carefully for major directions that it has not occurred to you to take. The pace of short memo writing ought to be especially great toward the beginning of your work. I would advocate the "idea" or "concept" memos that introduce an emerging idea. Such memos typically run two to three pages.*

Having reviewed our data and memos, we are now prepared to do what Karp terms "grabbing onto a theme" and create a *data memo*. This is memoing that consciously matches the theme we've chosen with specific data and literature that enforces what we've found. This becomes a more in-depth look at our data and ideas (later to be adapted into a paper) and offers the researcher a more precise and comprehensive way of examining all the data he or she has acquired to that point. Once again, as always, the researcher must continue to practice reflexivity and question whether he or she is accurately representing the respondents' stories and not the researcher's own viewpoint or bias. Continue memoing about this theme as well.

At this point, we also need to consider whether we will use a computer software data analysis program in our study. We discussed CAQDAS programs at length in Chapter 3, and I suggest you return to that chapter and its appendices to see what technology would aid your research project. Two main types of programs are specifically aimed at use in research. Generic software, not targeted for use in qualitative research, consists of word processors (to type and organize field notes and memos), text retrievers (to sort through data and identify patterns and themes within various data), and textbase managers (to retrieve semistructured information, used to structure "records" and "fields"; Fielding & Lee, 1998b).

The other types of software researchers can consider using are qualitative analysis packages, specifically designed for use in qualitative data analysis. This software comes in several forms as well: code-and-retrieve programs (assigning codes to text for easy later retrieval), code-based theory building programs (analyzing systematic relationships among data, codes, and categories), and conceptual network building and textual mapping software (drawing links between code categories; Fielding & Lee, 1998b, pp. 9–11). The best way to get to know these software programs and to identify which ones work with your research project is to experiment with them over time, getting to know their functions and applicability. Their growing popularity only increases research possibilities and aids functions for researchers.

---

### RESEARCH PRAXIS ASIDE 8. A USER-CENTERED APPROACH TO EMPLOYING COMPUTER-ASSISTED SOFTWARE TO ANALYZE MIXED METHODS DATA

The following set of reflective questions by Hesse-Biber and Crofts (2008, p. 665) are adapted partly from insights from Tesch (1990), Weitzman and Miles (1995), and Creswell and Maietta (2003), as well as Hesse-Biber and Crofts's (2008) own emphasis on issues regarding additional user-centered strategies that one might consider when thinking about purchasing and using a computer-assisted software program for analyzing data.

- What is my level of computer literacy? Do I consider myself a novice user, or, going to the opposite extreme, do I write my own computer programs?

- What type of computer system do I prefer to work on or feel most comfortable working on? Does the program support my operating system? Do I need to upgrade my system or perhaps purchase a new computer to meet the requirements of a specific program? Do I like the look and feel of a program's interface? What excites me about this program at a visceral level?

- Does the look and feel of the program fit with my own research style? What is my analysis style? How do I plan to conduct my analysis, and how might computers fit into that style? How might each program enhance (or detract from) my analysis? In what sense? Do I plan on coding most of my data? How do I prefer my data to be retrieved, and how important is it for me to be able to look at the full context from which the data were taken? Am I a visual person? Do I like to see relationships and concepts selected in some type of diagram or network? Do I anticipate quantifying any of my data?

- For what research project or set of projects do I anticipate using a computer software program? What types of data does my project consist of—textual or multimedia?

- How do I want a computer program to assist me? What tasks do I want to mechanize? What specific tasks do I want computerized? I may not want all the features contained in these programs. What are my expectations of what the program will be able to assist me in doing? Are my expectations realistic?

- What resources are available to me? Which programs can my computer support? Which programs can I afford? What resources (time, personnel, material) necessary for learning how to use this program are available to me?

- What are my preconceptions about these programs? How have other users' opinions, product marketing, or other sources of information about qualitative data analysis software programs influenced my preferences? Are my assumptions about programs accurate? What more would I like to learn about particular programs?

- Which of the preceding questions and concerns are most important to me? How would I rank-order my most important factors in considering a software purchase? What questions have been left out?

## Step 5. Writing Up a Mixed Methods Study

The writing up of this research project returns to the research question(s). We started out with the following questions:

- What is the lived experience of a male college football player?

- How do male college football players feel about their bodies?

- To what extent, if any, is the use of performance-enhancement drugs part of their experience as athletes?

- How prevalent is the use of performance-enhancement drugs and/or supplements among college football players? To what extent, if any, do they perceive it to be part of the lived experience of other college football players in general?

We would for the most part have a minimal integration of results from the analysis and interpretation in Phase 1. We might provide the reader with basic demographic results from Phase 1 by presenting some descriptive statistics on overall drug use among athletes gleaned from the survey. We would examine any statistically significant relationships that emerged from our analysis of the quantitative survey data and look for any differences by race and ethnicity. We would also present any social or psychological factors that ex-athletes mentioned most frequently as reasons that they might use enhancement drugs. Also, as we noted earlier, the findings from Phase 1 informed some of the questions for Phase 2, and within the conclusion section, we might begin by specifically integrating those findings from similar overlapping questions we asked in both studies. Phase 1 findings would still be considered as enhancing the more dominant presentation of the "main" findings from Phase 2, which would provide the reader with a sense of the range and depth of lived experiences of college athletes and would provide some dominant themes running through the in-depth interviews to characterize college athletes' experiences. The study would hopefully begin to generate some theoretical insights that would help the reader better understand an athlete's mind-set and the role of enhancement drugs in the everyday experience of college athletes. One major idea mentioned earlier was the process of normalization, and we might begin to see how this process plays out within the context of the interviews.

### RESEARCH PRAXIS ASIDE 9. QUESTIONS TO ASK AT THE WRITING-UP STAGE

An interesting issue to consider in a mixed methods write-up is the range of opportunities one may have missed to integrate research findings to get the most from a mixed methods study. In order to decide how well the study was run (or could have been run), consider these questions:

- Could I have integrated my findings at the data analysis stage? How and why?

- Could I have integrated my interpretations at the interpretation stage? How and why? Remember, integrating at the analysis and interpretation stage of a research project may or may not enhance one's understanding of the research problem.

In any research study, the researcher might have missed some valuable opportunities to add understanding to the overall project goals. Applying this to our specific example, we might point out that during the analysis of Phase 1, to what extent does the researcher use the findings to ask questions as Phase 2 proceeds? Were there issues or anomalies from Phase 1 that the researcher wanted to follow up with in Phase 2? For example, suppose Phase 1 uncovered unanticipated findings and found that not only were athletes using enhancement drugs but were also using a range of prescription drugs, as well as engaging in eating-disordered behaviors such as bulimia. To what extent does the researcher take these findings into account in terms of the focus of the research problem for Phase 2 and the types of questions they might ask and follow up on? To what extent does the researcher compare and contrast her or his analysis and interpretation, taking into account these and additional findings from Phase 1? By placing these two studies in conversation with one another, we can produce the synergy that is said to be characteristic of mixed methods designs. Yet, as we have seen in other studies, there remains very little integration at any stage in the mixed methods research process in general.

## RESEARCH PRAXIS ASIDE 10. TIPS TO WRITING UP A MIXED METHODS PROJECT: A HOLISTIC APPROACH

The writing process should be tightly linked to the research question(s) of the study. The research problem at hand should dictate the extent to which the findings of both methods are integrated and what the best mix should be. Your research problem should also determine how you present your research findings (analysis) and overall conclusions (interpretation). Several questions you should be contemplating during the writing process are:

- How will I specifically write up my analyses and interpretations from both studies?

- To what extent will I integrate my analyses and interpretations from each study?

- To what extent am I attentive to difference in my research findings? How will I deal with findings that are divergent?

Researchers must also remain consistent in practicing reflexivity during the writing stage of their mixed methods project. The following are guidelines to remember:

- Know your own standpoint as a researcher. What particular biases do you bring to or impose on your research? That means reflecting on your own assumptions about the nature of the social world (questions about ontology and epistemology).

- Examine your analytic biases. Are you wedded to one type of methods practice? Do you feel open to working with different methods and writing up research findings from multiple methods?

- Examine your methods skill level. Are you comfortable working with both qualitative and quantitative data? Are you knowledgeable about integrating mixed methods data?

- If you are working with a research team, has the research team reflected on how research findings will or will not be integrated? Remember that it will take social skills and time for research teams, especially with those who hold different assumptions about the nature of the social world, to work together.

# Conclusion:
# Evaluating Your Mixed Methods Project[2]

As we end this chapter, we provide you with the following checklist to consult as you begin your own research project. This list of questions is not exhaustive but is meant to highlight some of the important factors you might consider in undertaking your own evaluation of your research project as a whole.

- *Overall research question*

  **Ask**: Why should anyone "buy" my story? Why should anyone trust my story?

- *Issues of credibility*

  **Ask**: What are the set of criteria I should use in assessing the validity of my mixed methods project?

  **Ask**: Do I provide an "audit trail" of my work? Can the reader follow the analytical steps I provide as evidence of credibility?

- *Mixed methods design*

  **Ask**: Does my selected mixed methods research design fit my research problem?

  **Ask**: Is my method compatible with my purpose (research question)? How well versed am I in the data collection strategies described?

- *Sample*

  **Ask**: How were respondents chosen? Are these respondents a valid choice for this research?

- *Ethics*

  **Ask**: How are human participants' issues dealt with? Do I meet the standards of the IRB and my own ethical standards?

- *Analysis*

  **Ask**: How did I arrive at my specific findings?

  **Ask**: Why did I choose to mix or not mix data from my mixed methods project?

  **Ask**: Are specific analysis strategies talked about? Have I done what I said I would do?

  **Ask**: Are my different data analysis approaches compatible with my research question(s)?

- *Interpretation*

  **Ask**: Did I provide my reader with a sense (gestalt) of the meaning of the data from my written findings?

  **Ask**: Does the evidence fit my data? Are the data congruent with my research question(s)?

- *Conclusions/recommendations*

  **Ask**: Do conclusions reflect my research findings? Do I provide some recommendations for future research?

- *Significance of your work*

  **Ask**: What is the significance of my research? To what extent does my research offer a contribution to previous research in this area?

This chapter has illustrated how the iterative or back-and-forth process of mixed methods research is somewhat like fitting together the pieces of a puzzle. A few pieces of data can go a long way in gathering meaning, but one should not be tempted to gather too much data while failing to reflect on or analyze the information bit by bit. A creative spirit and a set of analytical and interpretative skills are imperative to this process. *Coding* and *memoing* are two powerful techniques we might employ in the process of understanding and interpreting our data; practicing reflexivity is also incredibly important. We may encounter false starts, as well as moments of great discovery and generation of theoretical insights into the analysis and interpretation of our data. This type of work is not for the fainthearted. It often requires an attention to detail, perseverance in the face of chaos, and a knack for tolerating ambiguity. The writing up of our research also requires that we, the researchers, be reflective of our own positionality—the set of social and economic attributes we bring to bear in analyzing and interpreting our data. It is a journey well worth taking, for it ultimately leads to a better understanding of the lived reality of those whom we research.

Our mixed methods journey is always bound to and guided by our researcher standpoint—those values and ethical concerns that extend beyond our own particular research projects. The research project is a site at which the personal and political merge. As this book comes to an end, we hope that it has been insightful, and we believe that the perspectives and tools we have provided you with will come in handy as you begin your own mixed methods research project.

Before ending this book, I return to what I believe is the promise of mixed methods research and also reflect on what issues mixed methods research still faces. In order to move forward in the application of mixed methods, we need to revise its promise, as well as the drawbacks researchers still confront in the practice of this method.

## APPENDIX 7.1. Examples of Consent Forms

### Consent Form Example 1

**Title of Research Project**: The Prevalence of Drug Use and Its Correlates among Ex-Football Athletes at Big Ten Universities: Phase 1

**Research Team**: [you would put your name and affiliation here]

**Contact Person**: [name, address, e-mail]

**To Whom It May Concern:**

I am a research sociologist who is heading a research team from both the Department of Sociology and the Department of Psychology at Boston College. We are undertaking a year-long project that seeks to ascertain the attitudes and behaviors of ex-college football players with regard to the range of motivations, pressures, and specific issues of college athletes, especially those who play or have played college football. We are especially interested in their perceptions of the frequency and range of use of performance-enhancing drugs.

We intend to conduct online surveys with all those first-string football players who have played football at a Big Ten University and who are now 1 to

5 years postcollege. We are contacting you now as your name is among those athletes who fit these sampling criteria, as taken from the pool of ex-football athletes whom we have identified from a range of sources, including sports archives at your former university and ads we have placed on various sports-related websites.

We hope that you will agree to take part in our study, which involves completing the e-mail survey attached to this e-mail. If you choose to participate, please indicate your agreement to participate by printing out this letter and placing an "X" in the square box below. Please fill out the survey that is also attached to this e-mail. E-mail both these separate attachments to the e-mail address under the heading "contact person" at the top of this e-mail letter. Do not sign your name on either the consent form or questionnaire, in order to ensure confidentiality of your survey.

The findings from our study will be valuable in our seeking to understand how to best serve the needs and concerns of college athletes. Your participation is voluntary, and if you have any questions about our project, feel free to contact a member of our research team listed at the top of this e-mail.

\*\*\*\*\*\*\*\*\*\*\*\*\*\*\*\*\*\*\*\*\*\*\*\*\*\*\*\*\*\*\*\*\*\*\*\*\*\*\*\*\*\*\*\*\*\*\*\*\*\*\*\*\*\*\*\*\*\*\*\*\*

**I consent to participate in this study.**   ☐

**Check the box to indicate your consent.**

**Consent date:** _____

## Consent Form Example 2

**Research Title:** The Experience of Being a College Football Athlete

**To Whom It May Concern:**

I am a research sociologist at Boston College, Chestnut Hill, Massachusetts. I am heading up a research project whose goal is to understand the experience of being a starting-string football player at a Big Ten university. This is the second part of the study; the first phase consisted of a survey of a random sample of college football players at Big Ten universities that looked at the larger set of motivations and attitudes for playing football and the range of specific issues and problems athletes confront in college. Phase 2 of our study seeks to interview former football players in depth to get a sense of their lived experience in being a football player in terms of their personal perspective on combining athletics with academics and the challenges they may confront in doing so. We also are interested in their perceptions of the use, if any, of performance-enhancing drugs in college athletics.

The interview will be tape-recorded over the phone. Your participation is completely voluntary. The interview is confidential, and only our research team will see your interview. We intend to collate our results without any identifying information. These data will be written up for publication, as well as for presentations at conferences.

It is our hope that your information will help benefit and enhance the college experience of athletes both in their sports and in their academic lives. Please reply to this e-mail by pressing the "reply" button and letting us know when we might contact you for an interview by placing a checkmark on all dates and times you are available during the week. Additionally, please check the boxes below so that we might gauge your eligibility for this study. We hope to hear from you soon. Thanks!

\*\*\*\*\*\*\*\*\*\*\*\*\*\*\*\*\*\*\*\*\*\*\*\*\*\*\*\*\*\*\*\*\*\*\*\*\*\*\*\*\*\*\*\*\*\*\*\*\*\*\*\*\*\*\*\*

**I consent to participate in this study.**  ☐

**Check box to indicate your consent.**

**Consent date:** _____

**I am available for contact on these days and times.**

**Mon.**_____   **Tues.**_____   **Wed.**_____

**Thurs.**_____   **Fri.**_____   **Sat.**_____

**Fill out the specific time(s) you can be reached by phone in the line next to each day.**

## GLOSSARY

**data memo:** memos that connect themes discovered by the researcher to specific data and literature that reinforce the findings.

**focused coding:** a process that looks at all the data that has been coded and creates more interpretative and inclusive codes to represent an understanding of what respondents say.

**narrative analysis:** a researcher looks at data as a whole, concentrating on how the subject's narrative is told.

**normalization:** process by which a behavior or idea is made to seem "normal" through repetition until it is taken for granted.

**praxis:** a practice exercise for the application of a theory (e.g., a practice research project to apply qualitative mixed methods).

DISCUSSION QUESTIONS

1. Cite some specific research problems that lend themselves to a mixed methods approach and explain why.

2. What are the steps involved in conducting a mixed methods project?

3. What rule does reflexivity play in carrying out a mixed methods project?

■ ■ ■ SUGGESTED WEBSITES ■ ■ ■

### Method and Research Design

*www.languages.ait.ac.th/el21meth.htm*

This is an interactive website on method and research design.

### Data Collection

*www.sagepub.com/upm-data/10983_Chapter_6.pdf*

This chapter from the book *Designing and Conducting Mixed Methods Research* by John W. Creswell and Vicki L. Plano Clark discusses data collection in mixed methods research.

### Data Analysis

*www.analytictech.com/borgatti/qualqua.htm*

This website discusses a type of mixed methods research in which qualitative data is analyzed via quantitative methodology, coding in particular.

### Mixed Methods Research

*www.osra.org/itlpj/roccoblissgallagherperez-pradospring2003.pdf*

This article gives a history of mixed methods research, different ways of thinking within mixed methods, purposes for using a mixed methods design, and eight types of mixed methods studies. The authors also analyze three specific studies and describe the benefits of mixed methods to organizational systems.

## NOTES

1. This section is adapted from Hesse-Biber and Leavy (2006a). Copyright 2006 by Sage Publications, Inc. Adapted by permission.

2. This section is adapted from Hesse-Biber and Leavy (2006a). Copyright 2006 by Sage Publications, Inc. Adapted by permission.

# CHAPTER 8

# Conclusion

## The Prospects and Challenges
## of Mixed Methods Praxis

W e hope this book inspires you to explore the paradigm shift implicit in the comprehensive approach to mixed methods research. We end our journey with a mixed methods tale that embodies the prospects and challenges of this method.

## A Mixed Methods Tale

Many think of ovarian cancer as a "silent killer," but experts now believe there are symptoms at its earliest stages that hold out promise of early detection. The following is an excerpt from an article taken from WebMD, a medical information website:

> Doctors used to call ovarian cancer "the silent killer." That's because it was thought to have no symptoms until the very late stages of disease. But women who had or who survived ovarian cancer insisted that they knew something was wrong, long before doctors finally diagnosed their malignancy.
>
> Finally, a doctor listened. University of Washington researcher Barbara Goff, MD, and colleagues analyzed patients' complaints and, in a groundbreaking 2004 study, announced to the medical world that ovarian cancer is not silent.

In 2007, Goff, M. Robyn Andersen, Ph.D., of Fred Hutchinson Cancer Research Center, and colleagues came up with a "symptom index" indicative of ovarian cancer. But this index caught only 57% of early-stage cancers.

Now the same researchers find that by adding a blood test for the CA125 ovarian-cancer biomarker—which by itself misses about half of ovarian cancers—the symptom index can catch more than four out of five early ovarian cancers.

"The symptom index and the CA125 test each finds 50% to 60% of women with early disease," Andersen tells WebMD. "But when they're combined, if either one is positive, we might be able to identify 80% of women with early stage ovarian cancer. Women with early stage disease have good chance of a cure—it's just that right now, we don't find many of them in time." (DeNoon, 2008, p. 1)

Such a monumental change in the perception of ovarian cancer makes one wonder how exactly the doctors and researchers were able to discover these previously unknown symptoms. What caused this turnabout in the diagnosis of ovarian cancer?

By listening to and taking seriously survivors' experiences, medical experts were able to piece together some important early warning signs of ovarian cancer, such as bloating or increased abdominal size, abdominal pain, and difficulty eating. Prior to this novel approach to diagnosis, women who expressed symptoms of ovarian cancer in its early stage found their symptoms easily dismissed or misdiagnosed by their physicians as typical "female disorders," such as eating disorders, depression, or anxiety.

Diagnosticians of ovarian cancer, however, discovered that the so-called "silent killer" has a voice. By employing a qualitative approach, which included listening carefully to patients' symptoms and analyzing their accounts, a clear pattern of early-warning signs emerged. A qualitative diagnosis then served as an important new diagnostic *symptom index* for early detection of ovarian cancer. Furthermore, the combination of these accounts with more quantitative methods, such as blood tests, provided a synergy that resulted in dramatic increases in the early detection of ovarian cancer to 80% (Goff et al., 2007, p. 224).

This development in the diagnosis of ovarian cancer demonstrates the promise of employing a mixed methods approach for more fully understanding the onset of a life-threatening disease. It also brings to the forefront the importance of introducing new methodological perspectives that break down entrenched ways of thinking about a given issue or problem. In this case, the *medical paradigm,* with its focus on objective diagnostic criteria (e.g., a blood test for a protein associated with ovarian cancer, a transvaginal ultrasound, and exploratory surgery) is challenged by a new way of thinking about diagnosis that includes listening seriously to patients' accounts of their symptoms, leading to an integration of mind and body into the diagnostic medical evaluation (DeNoon, 2008, p. 2).

This story also underscores the contributions that a *mixed methodological approach* can offer in shedding light on a complex problem. The successful result of the "ovarian cancer symptoms" research project is an acknowledgment of patient expertise about their own bodies and the importance of qualitative approaches that center subjective experience and participant voices. It also reveals the partial knowledge of medical diagnostic procedures that primarily rely on a positivist paradigm wedded to objective measures. It was the combination of the two methodological approaches, along with being open to mixing methods of diagnosis, that allowed this breakthrough in diagnosing ovarian cancer in its curable stages. How did Dr. Barbara Goff and her colleagues make this breakthrough?

In an interview with the *Ladies' Home Journal*, Barbara A. Goff, MD, Director of Gynecologic Oncology at the University of Washington, described her breakthrough diagnosis discovery. It is clear from her description that her decision to use a qualitative approach to diagnosis in addition to more standard clinical evidence was based on her perception that patients' own experiences and self-observations could be a significant and reliable indicator of disease—evidence that is typically discounted in traditional medical approaches to cancer diagnosis: "I was impressed by the ease with which these women could recall the health problems that preceded their diagnosis. . . . So many had been significantly blown off when they tried to talk to their doctors. Then they ended up having ovarian cancer after all" (quoted in Winters, 2007).

Dr. Goff went on to describe how difficult it was to obtain funding for her "patient symptoms" study and that most of her research was done on a "shoestring" budget, with some of the monies actually donated by her patients: "A patient donated $1,000 to cover research costs, and a statistician donated her time, while [patient Cindy] Melancon came up with a mailing list. 'We found that 97 percent of the 1,700 women in the study reported symptoms prior to their diagnosis'" (Winters, 2007).[1]

It took "doggedness and persistence" on the part of Dr. Goff, noted one ovarian cancer survivor. "'As people who had ovarian cancer, we knew there were symptoms in the early stages. Dr. Goff listened. That wasn't the case with many physicians' " (quoted in Winters, 2007).

It is clear from this example and from previous chapters in this book that a qualitatively driven approach to mixed methods, when implemented in a thoughtful manner that is driven by both theory and the research problem at hand, can add much to our understanding of complex research topics. Yet there remain misunderstandings and barriers to the practice of mixed methods. We revisit some of the most important of these next.

## Confusing Methodology with Method

Mixed methods research is not about creating a new methods paradigm. The rush to create mixed methods templates and elaborate systems of combining methods without paying attention to how various methods relate to research problems and methodologies have the effect of turning the study of mixed methods into a techniques-driven enterprise that promises more than it can deliver. Methods are tools that collect and analyze data and should be considered "a-theoretical and a-methodological" (Giddings & Grant, 2006, p. 4).

In Danish writer Hans Christian Andersen's 1837 tale, *The Emperor's New Clothes*, swindlers trick the emperor into believing he is wearing fine garments that are only visible to those who are wise like himself. In fact, he is clothed only in his underwear. All who come into contact with the emperor praise his fine clothing, lest they be taken for fools, unfit for public office.

The story of the emperor's clothes provides a cautionary tale for mixed methods practice. Although it is commonly assumed that there is inherent synergy in a mixed methods project, that the whole is greater than the sum of its parts, and that mixing qualitative and quantitative research makes for a better study, the simple deployment of these techniques without consideration of their relevance to the research problem will not necessarily yield the expected results. Likewise, pretending that the emperor is wearing clothing does not necessarily make his regal clothing a reality. Like the emperor's new clothes, the promise of a mixed methods design may be an illusion if it is practiced in an uninformed manner. In the past 5 years, the field of mixed methods research has witnessed a gold-rush mentality—frenzied activity on the part of a range of researchers seeking to jump on the mixed methods bandwagon. Janice Morse captured this frantic endeavor, reflecting on her observations of the development of mixed methods practice:

> I watch with interest the emergence of mixed-method design, and the inconsistency and lack of agreement over something as simple and straightforward as terminology. I look at the mixed method design scramble, with researchers competing to publish (and thereby attach their name to) the best taxonomy of mixed-methods designs. And some designs look so nonsensical to me that I am certain that the developers have never gotten their hands dirty and actually tried to do mixed methods themselves. (Morse, 2006, pp. 3–4)

Even this gold-rush mentality in the field of mixed methods cannot possibly capture the range of mixed methods designs, given especially the innovative nature of qualitative approaches to mixed methods that often encourages serendipity and openness across the research process.

Undertaking a qualitative approach to mixed methods is like taking a journey without always being in control of your destination. The book, *Qualitative Research and Evaluation Methods,* by Michael Quinn Patton (2002), an expert in the field of evaluation research, has become a benchmark. Patton was recently interviewed as part of a series, "The Oral History of Evaluation," by the Oral History Team Project for the *American Journal of Evaluation* (Oral History Project Team, 2007). Patton reflected on his research methods journey, and his remarks remind us that it is often the journey itself that leads to the discovery of ideas. Patton spent a great deal of his time hiking in the Grand Canyon and compared his experiences to his research work. In fact, he wrote a book about his personal experiences titled *Grand Canyon Celebration* (Patton, 1999). Here, he discussed how he views his experiences of hiking in the Grand Canyon as a metaphor for evaluation research:

> The most powerful experiences I've had in the Canyon have been what complexity scientists would call emergent experiences that you couldn't set out to try to have because you don't even know they exist. The people who are changing the world in major ways are often those kinds of people. They aren't the performance measurement people or the performance targets people. That orientation works well for evaluating immunization campaigns, but we don't know how to immunize people against poverty and social injustice. The people who are operating out of vision, social innovators who are learning

to pay attention to their environment and what's going on around them and acting responsively, they want the rigor of evaluative thinking that developmental evaluation offers, but without the baggage of forced, imposed, and premature clear, specific, and measurable objectives. (Oral History Project Team, 2007, p. 114)

Michael Patton's remarks remind us of the necessity to think outside our disciplinary methodology and to seek out *emergent experiences* that allow the discovery process to take root. Researchers should also use any experiences, ideas, and tools that can facilitate this process.

## The Importance of Emergent Methods for Mixed Methods Research

Mixed methods is part of a larger umbrella term, *emergent methods,* that refers to the new and alternative methods tools that arise from *emergent technologies* such as global positioning systems (GPS), the Internet and its applications, and new technologies of the future, such as developing nanotechnologies. *Nanotechnologies* are those technological developments at the atomic level that hold great promise of providing new emergent tools to the researcher for exploring previously unresearchable questions and opening up areas of uncharted research inquiry (Ebbesen, 2008). "Emergent methods" also refers to the use of traditional methods tools in new ways (Hesse-Biber & Leavy, 2006d). The mixing of traditional methods is an example of how researchers can reinscribe traditional tools, combining them into a range of new mixed methods research designs.

The demand for emergent methods also comes from those researchers now working in interdisciplinary research contexts in which the mixing of methodologies may often require new methods to tackle innovative ideas that come from this type of collaboration. From an emergent methods perspective, mixed methods, although an important innovation, is one of the many tools yet to be thoroughly explored and practiced by social researchers. An overreliance on certain methods and an unexamined belief in their promises may serve to limit researchers' ability to answer new and complex issues and problems.

Emergent methods in the end are tools, and what matters is the overarching awareness on the part of the researcher that all tools must be placed in their research context.

# The Challenges of Utilizing
# a Mixed Methods Approach

There remain significant challenges in practicing mixed methods that involve issues of training, philosophical and disciplinary barriers, funding limitations, and additional roadblocks that may limit the publication of mixed methods research.

Mixed methods practice and pedagogy needs to be open to a range of innovations in methods and not to be too quick to create specific templates for mixed methods designs that may lead to a form of mixed methods orthodoxy. The number of textbooks and articles devoted to the topic of mixed methods research has grown dramatically, and many of these provide "cookbook" approaches to mixed methods design and deal with permutations and combinations of mixing both quantitative and qualitative methods—from the timing and sequence of these methods to discussions of what methods should be primary or secondary in one's analysis.

One challenge lies in overcoming a "methods experience gap." Using mixed methods requires training in and knowledge of both quantitative and qualitative methods, but most researchers have expertise with only one method. The uneven knowledge and application of methods can negatively affect the research process; and if the researcher is unable to successfully use both methods, the integrity of a mixed methods project may be compromised.

In addition to an inability to implement both methods, another challenge comes with attempting to deal with different *epistemological* and *methodological standpoints*. We have already discussed that researchers need to be aware of their own research standpoints at all stages of the research process and that in order to conduct mixed methods research, researchers need to step out of their comfort zones, both in terms of the methods they use and the view of nature and reality from which they are working. This brings up the need for *reflexivity*, prompting researchers to contemplate their particular agendas and how they can successfully cross disciplinary boundaries and mix methods.

Academic traditions also pose a challenge for mixed methods research. Departmental culture is a powerful influence on the choice of methods that are practiced. Both the influence of colleagues on one another's research and the influence of professors on students' research techniques can lead to the favoring of a certain set of methods. Green and Preston (2005) referred to this circumstance as "specialisms" whereby "university faculties and departments are . . . 'oriented' towards a particular qualitative or quantitative research specialism (or groups of specialisms)" (p. 168). This is, for example, how qualitative methods came to define and form the Chicago School of Sociology in the 1920s, though quantitative research was also being performed there (Platt, 1996). Department training programs may not provide training in both qualitative and quantitative methods, and even fewer may have courses in mixed methods. These pressures toward specialism can extend to other knowledge builders, publishers of social research, and social policy makers who may be wedded to one type of methods reporting—qualitative or quantitative, but not both.

As mentioned earlier in this book, the pressure to specialize in one method or the other can also come from funding agencies. Some funding agencies may suggest or support a particular research method, and the individual researcher feels compelled to comply with their preferences in order to get support. Just as the researcher has an agenda or specific point of view from which he or she operates, so too do funding agencies. Alvin Gouldner (1970) believes that funding agencies negatively influence the methodology of sociological research and attributes their influence to the growth of "theoryless" theories (p. 44). According to Gouldner, a "utilitarian culture" has grown up around the practice of social research that "always tends towards a theoryless empiricism in which the conceptualization of problems is secondary and energies are instead given over to questions of measurement, research or experimental design, sampling or instrumentation" (Gouldner, 1970, p. 82). However, other researchers feel that this explanation gives funding agencies too much credit and blame other factors, such as departmental cultures, for the denial of funds for mixed methods projects (see Platt, 1996).

These various challenges to mixed methods approaches, if they are to be overcome, require new practices and an awareness and application of new methods. Working in an interdisciplinary manner takes researchers out of their comfort zones and requires good communication, because different fields come with their own epistemologies. When working in research teams, as is increasingly happening, particularly in interdisciplinary studies, a multitude of views (research paradigms) are present, and researchers need to discuss and incorporate all of their epistemological views into their approach. The more open researchers are to incorporating new ideas, the more possibilities they have to choose from when deciding on their research projects. Additionally, they can decide which characteristics of different methods are most useful for the project at hand. Interdisciplinary teamwork has its unique challenges. Klein (1990) reminded us that because of the differences between disciplines and the number of disciplines one can integrate in a study, there exists a potential for communication problems in interdisciplinary teamwork (p. 183).

In an interview with Julianne Cheek, a leading postmodern social researcher, we talked about what advice she would give to novice researchers who are thinking about a mixed methods approach:

> *The advice I give to my own students is to work out why you're doing what you're doing and why you want to do what you're doing. . . . In addition, my advice would be to remember that methods are theoretical and to remember that methodology is theoretical and then remember that you've got theoretical frames that sit above that. . . . It's not just technicians that we want. It is researchers. And research is much more than the technical exercise of collecting the data.*

## The Need for a Comprehensive Approach to Mixed Methods

This book takes a comprehensive approach to the practice of mixed methods that places the research question as the primary force in understanding the development of mixed methods designs from collection to analysis, interpretation, and writing up of findings. This approach asks:

- What are the specific advantages and disadvantages of using a mixed methods approach?

- What particular research problems and methodologies lend themselves to mixing methods?

- What specific research designs and analyses might flow from these methodologies?

- How and at what stage in the process of a research project should methods be mixed, if at all?

We focus on qualitative approaches to mixed methods research and stress the importance of a multivocal understanding of social reality that gets at the subjective experiences of the researched. This is a generative model of understanding a social reality that is open, expansive, and subject to revision. The practice of a qualitative approach to mixed methods research is not necessarily linear but rather in a constant state of flux, changing in response to research findings and revision of research questions. It utilizes both quantitative and qualitative methods in the service of its research agenda. It does not stop at asking what a qualitative investigation can do to enhance a quantitative study, nor does it seek to use qualitative methods solely as a preliminary source of data for creating new questions to include on a survey. A qualitative approach does not seek solely to serve as a means to explain unexpected findings in a quantitative study or to evaluate the impact of an intervention or outcome, as it has been primarily used in the past.

The analysis of mixed methods data seeks, where applicable to the research question, to place the findings from both qualitative and quantitative data in conversation—perhaps to test out ideas or even reformulate a research problem. A qualitative approach to mixed methods research is particularly relevant to social justice goals because it seeks to uncover subjugated knowledge and exposes inequities within society by challenging dominant views of reality.

A qualitative approach is not about the method, it is about methodology—theoretical perspectives onto social realities. For too long, mixed methods approaches have added qualitative methods to fundamentally quantitative methodologies in a way that does not do justice to the power and potential of a qualitative approach.

Let's begin to change this.

## GLOSSARY

**emergent experiences:** experiences that occur unexpectedly and allow new discoveries.

**emergent methods:** new and alternative tools that arise from new technologies such as global positioning systems (GPS) and developing technologies such as nanotechnology, or the use of traditional methods in new ways.

---

## DISCUSSION QUESTIONS

1. What is the distinction between method and methodology?

2. What is meant by the "methods experience gap"?

3. What are some challenges of utilizing a mixed methods approach?

---

## ■ ■ ■ SUGGESTED WEBSITE ■ ■ ■

*personal.bgsu.edu/~earlem/MIXEDMETHODS/*

This is a special interest website that is a forum for researchers who are interested in "conducting, designing, teaching, and advancing issues related to the appropriate mixing of qualitative and quantitative methods in research" (from the website's description).

## NOTE

1. All excerpts from Winters (2007). Copyright 2007 by Meredith Corporation. First published in *Ladies' Home Journal*. Reprinted by permission.

# References

Acquisti, A., & Gross, R. (2006). Imagined communities: Awareness, information sharing and privacy on the Facebook. In P. Golle & G. Danezis (Eds.), *Proceedings of the 6th Workshop on Privacy Enhancing Technologies* (pp. 36–58). Cambridge, UK: Robinson College.

Agger, B. (1991). Critical theory, poststructuralism, postmodernism: Their sociological relevance. *Annual Review of Sociology, 17*, 105–131.

Agger, B. (1998). *Critical social theories: An introduction.* Boulder, CO: Westview Press.

Anderson, L. (2006). Analytic autoethnography. *Journal of Contemporary Ethnography, 35*(4), 373–395.

Andrews, D., Nonnecke, B., & Preece, J. (2003). Electronic survey methodology: A case study in reaching hard-to-involve Internet users. *International Journal of Human–Computer Interaction, 16*(2), 185–210.

Bahl, S., & Milne, G. R. (2006). Mixed methods in interpretative research: An application to the study of the self concept. In R. W. Belk (Ed.), *The handbook of qualitative research methods in marketing* (pp. 198–218). Cheltenham, UK: Edward Elgar.

Bailey, C. (1996). *A guide to field research.* Thousand Oaks, CA: Pine Forge Press.

Banks, J. A. (1976). Comment on "A content analysis of the black American in textbooks." In M. P. Golden (Ed.), *The research experience* (pp. 383–389). Itasca, IL: Peacock.

Bergman, M. A. (Ed.). (2008). *Advances in mixed methods research.* London: Sage.

Bertens, H. (1995). *The idea of the postmodern: A history.* London: Routledge.

Bhavnani, K. (1993). Tracing the contours: Feminist research and feminist objectivity. *Women's Studies International Forum, 16*, 95–104.

Body image: Equal-opportunity anxiety. (2002, November). *Tufts University Health and Nutrition Letter, 20*(9), 1.

Booth, C. (1892–1897). *Life and labour of the people in London.* London: Macmillan.

Bowker, N. I. (2001). Understanding online communities through multiple methodologies combined under a postmodern research endeavour. *Forum Qualitative Sozialforschung/Forum: Qualitative Social Research, 2*(1). Available at *www.qualitative-research.net/fqs-texte/1-01/1-01bowker-e.htm.*

Bowles, G., & Duelli Klein, R. (Eds.). (1983). *Theories of women's studies.* London: Routledge & Kegan Paul.

Boyd, D., & Ellison, N. (2007). Social network sites: Definition, history and scholarship. *Journal of Computer-Mediated Communication, 13*(1), 210–230.

Brannen, J. (2005, December). *Mixed methods research: A discussion paper* (Economic and Social Research Council National Centre for Research Methods Review Papers). Available at *www.ncrm.ac.uk/research/outputs/publications/documents/MethodsReviewPaperNCRM-005.pdf.*

Brannen, J., Dodd, K., Oakley, A., & Storey, P. (1994). *Young people, health and family life.* Philadelphia: Open University Press.

Brewer, J. D., & Hunter, A. (1989). *Multimethod research: A synthesis of styles.* Newbury Park, CA: Sage.

Brown, L. M., & Gilligan, C. (1992). *Meeting at the crossroads: Women's psychology and girls' development.* Cambridge, MA: Harvard University Press.

Bruce, C. (2007). CIA gets in your Face(book). *Wired.* Available at *www.wired.com/techbiz/it/news/2007/01/72545.*

Bryman, A. (1988). *Quantity and quality in social research.* New York: Routledge.

Bryman, A. (2006). Integrating quantitative and qualitative research: How is it done? *Qualitative Research, 6,* 97–113.

Bryman, A. (2007a). Barriers to integrating quantitative and qualitative research. *Journal of Mixed Methods Research, 1*(1), 8–22.

Bryman, A. (2007b). The research question in social research: What is its role? *International Journal of Social Research Methodology, 10*(1), 5–20.

Bryman, A. (2008). Why do researchers integrate/combine/mesh/blend/mix/merge/fuse quantitative and qualitative research? In M. M. Bergman (Ed.), *Advances in mixed methods research,* (pp. 89–100). London: Sage.

Bulmer, M. (1984). *The Chicago School of sociology: Institutionalization, diversity, and the rise of sociological research.* Chicago: University of Chicago Press.

Charmaz, K. (1983). The grounded theory method: An explication and interpretation. In R. M. Emerson (Ed.), *Contemporary field research: A collection of readings* (pp. 109–126). Prospect Heights, IL: Waveland Press.

Charmaz, K. (1995). Grounded theory. In J. Smith, R. Harrow, & L. Van Langenhove (Eds.), *Rethinking methods in psychology* (pp. 27–49). London: Sage.

Cheek, J. (1999). Influencing practice or simply esoteric?: Researching health care using postmodern approaches. *Qualitative Health Research, 9*(3), 383–392.

Cheek, J. (2000). *Postmodern and poststructural approaches to nursing research.* Thousand Oaks, CA: Sage.

Cisneros-Puebla, C. A. (2004). Let's do more theoretical work: Janice Morse in conversation with Cesar A. Cisneros-Puebla. *Forum Qualitative Sozialforschung (Form: Qualitative Social Research), 5*(3). Available at *www.qualitative-research.net/fqs-texte/3-04/04-3-33-e.htm.*

Cohane, G. H., & Pope, H. G. (2001). Body image in boys: A review of the literature. *International Journal of Eating Disorders, 29*(4), 373–379.

Cohen, J. (1988). *Statistical power analysis for the behavioral sciences* (2nd ed.). Hillsdale, NJ: Erlbaum.

Collins, K. M. T., Onwuegbuzie, A. J., & Jiao, Q. G. (2006). Prevalence of mixed methods sampling designs in social science research. *Evaluation and Research in Education, 19*(2), 83–101.

Collins, K. M. T., Onwuegbuzie, A. J., & Jiao, Q. G. (2007). A mixed methods investigation of mixed methods sampling designs in social and health science research. *Journal of Mixed Methods Research, 1*(3), 267–294.

Collins, P. H. (2000). *Black feminist thought: Knowledge, consciousness, and the politics.* Boston: Unwin Hyman.

Crabtree, B. F., & Miller, W. L. (1999). *Doing qualitative research.* Thousand Oaks, CA: Sage.

Creswell, J. (1998). *Quality inquiry and research design: Choosing among five traditions.* Thousand Oaks, CA: Sage.

Creswell, J. (2003). *Research design: Qualitative, quantitative, and mixed methods approaches* (1st ed.). Thousand Oaks, CA: Sage.

Creswell, J. (2006). *Qualitative inquiry and research design: Choosing among five approaches* (2nd ed.). Thousand Oaks, CA: Sage.

Creswell, J. (2008). *Research design: Qualitative, quantitative and mixed methods approaches* (3rd ed.). Thousand Oaks, CA: Sage.

Creswell, J. W., & Maietta, R. C. (2003). Qualitative research. In D. C. Miller & N. J. Salkind (Eds.), *Handbook of research design and social measurement* (pp. 143–200). Thousand Oaks, CA: Sage.

Creswell, J. W., & Plano Clark, V. L. (2008). *Designing and conducting mixed methods research.* Thousand Oaks, CA: Sage.

Creswell, J. W., Plano Clark, V. L., Gutmann, M., & Hanson, W. (2003). Advanced mixed methods research designs. In A. Tashakkori & C. Teddlie (Eds.), *Handbook of mixed methods in social and behavioral research* (pp. 209–240). Thousand Oaks, CA: Sage.

Creswell, J. W., Shope, R., Plano Clark, V. L., & Green, D. O. (2006). How interpretive qualitative research extends mixed methods research. *Research in the Schools, 13*(1), 1–11.

Deleuze, G., & Guattari, F. (1987). *A thousand plateaus: Capitalism and schizophrenia.* London: Athlone Press.

DeNoon, D. J. (2008, June 23). Symptoms warn of ovarian cancer. *WebMD Health News.* Available at *www.webmd.com/ovarian cancer/news/20080623/symptoms-warn-of-ovarian-cancer.*

Denzin, N. (2001). *Interpretive interactionism.* Thousand Oaks, CA: Sage.

Denzin, N. K., & Lincoln, Y. S. (Eds.). (1998). *Collecting and interpreting qualitative materials.* Thousand Oaks, CA: Sage.

Derrida, J. (1966). The decentering event and social thought. In *Writing and difference* (A. Bass, Trans.; pp. 278–282). Chicago: University of Chicago Press.

Dobb, A. N., & Gross, A. E. (1976). Status of frustrator as an inhibitor of horn-honking responses. In M. P. Golden (Ed.), *The research experience* (pp. 481–494). Itasca, IL: Peacock.

Ebbesen, M. (2008). The role of the humanities and social sciences in nanotechnology research and development. *NanoEthics, 2*(1), 1–13.

Ely, M., Vinz, R., Anzul, M., & Downing, M. (1999). *On writing qualitative research: Living by words* (2nd ed.). London: Falmer.

Fielding, N., & Lee, R. (1998a). *Computer analysis and qualitative research*. London: Sage.

Fielding, N., & Lee, R. (1998b). Introduction: Computer analysis and qualitative research. In N. Fielding & R. Lee (Eds.), *Computer analysis and qualitative research* (pp. 1–20). London: Sage.

Fine, M. (1988). Sexuality, schooling, and adolescent females: The missing discourse of desire. *Harvard Educational Review, 58*(1), 29–53.

Foucault, M. (1975). *Discipline and punish: The birth of the prison* (A. Sheridan, Trans.). New York: Vintage Books.

Frost, M. (1999). Health visitors' perceptions of domestic violence: The private nature of the problem. *Journal of Advanced Nursing, 30*(3), 589–596.

Gannon, S., & Davies, B. (2007). Postmodern, poststructural, and critical theories. In S. Nagy Hesse-Biber (Ed.), *Handbook of feminist research: Theory and praxis* (pp. 71–106). Thousand Oaks, CA: Sage.

Gerbert, B., Abercrombie, P., Caspers, N., Love, C., & Bronstone, A. (1999). How health care providers help battered women: The survivor's perspective. *Women and Health, 29*(3), 115–135.

Giddings, L. S. (2006). Mixed-methods research: Positivism dressed in drag? *Journal of Research in Nursing, 11*(3), 195–203.

Giddings, L. S., & Grant, B. M. (2006). Mixed methods for the novice researcher. *Contemporary Nurse, 23*, 3–11.

Giddings, L. S., & Grant, B. M. (2007). A Trojan horse for positivism?: A critique of mixed methods research. *Advances in Nursing Science, 30*(1), 52–60.

Gilgun, J. (1992). Hypothesis generation in social work research. *Journal of Social Service Research, 15*(3/4), 113–135.

Gilgun, J. F. (1999). Methodological pluralism and qualitative family research. In M. Sussman, S. K. Steinmetz, & G. W. Peterson (Eds.), *Handbook of marriage and the family* (2nd ed., pp. 219–261). New York: Plenum Press.

Gilgun, J. F., Klein, C., & Pranis, K. (2000). The significance of resources in models of risk. *Journal of Interpersonal Violence, 15*(6), 631–650.

Glaser, B., & Strauss, A. L. (1967). *The discovery of grounded theory: Strategies for qualitative research*. Chicago: Aldine.

Goff, B. A., Mandel, L. S., Drescher, C. W., Urban, N., Gough, S., Schurman, K. M., et al. (2007). Development of an ovarian cancer symptom index. *Cancer, 109*(2), 221–227.

Gouldner, A. W. (1970). *The coming crisis of Western sociology*. New York: Basic Books.

Green, A., & Preston, J. (2005). Speaking in tongues: Diversity in mixed methods research *[Editorial]. International Journal of Social Research Methodology, 8*(3), 167–171.

Green, G., Uryasz, F., Petr, T., & Bray, D. (2001). NCAA study of substance use and abuse habits of college student athletes. *Clinical Journal of Sport Medicine, 11*(1), 51–56.

Greene, J. C. (2002). With a splash of soda, please: Towards active engagement with difference. *Evaluation, 8*(2), 259–266.

Greene, J. C. (2007). *Mixed methods in social inquiry*. San Francisco: Jossey-Bass.

Greene, J. C., Benjamin, L., & Goodyear, L. (2001). The merits of mixing methods in evaluation. *Evaluation, 7*, 25–44.

Greene, J. C., & Caracelli, V. J. (Eds.). (1997). *Advances in mixed-method evaluation: The challenges and benefits of integrating diverse paradigms. New Directions for Evaluation, 74.* San Francisco: Jossey-Bass.

Greene, J. C., Caracelli, V. J., & Graham, W. F. (1989). Toward a conceptual framework for mixed-method evaluation designs. *Educational Evaluation and Policy Analysis, 11*(3), 255–274.

Grim, B. J., Harmon, A. H., & Gromis, J. C. (2006). Focused group interviews as an innovative quanti-qualitative methodology (QQM): Integrating quantitative elements into a qualitative methodology. *Qualitative Report, 11*(3), 516–537.

Guba, E. G., & Lincoln, Y. S. (1994). Competing paradigms in research. In N. K. Denzin & Y. S. Lincoln (Eds.), *Handbook of qualitative research* (pp. 105–107). Thousand Oaks, CA: Sage.

Gubrium, J. F., & Holstein, J. A. (1997). *The new language of qualitative method.* New York: Oxford University Press.

Gustafson-Larson, A. M., & Terry, R. D. (1992). Weight-related behaviors and concerns of fourth-grade children. *Journal of the American Dietetic Association, 18*, 199–126.

Hanson, W. E., Creswell, J. W., Plano Clark, V. L., Petska, K. S., & Creswell, J. D. (2005). Mixed methods research designs in counseling psychology. *Journal of Counseling Psychology, 52*(2), 224–235.

Haraway, D. (1988). Situated knowledges: The science question in feminism and the privilege of partial perspectives. *Feminist Studies, 14*(13), 575–599.

Harding, S. G. (Ed.). (1987). *Feminism and methodology.* Bloomington: Indiana University Press.

Harding, S. G. (1991). *Whose science? Whose knowledge?* Ithaca, NY: Cornell University Press.

Harding, S. G. (1993). Rethinking standpoint epistemology: "What is strong objectivity?" In L. Alcoff & E. Potter (Eds.), *Feminist epistemologies* (pp. 49–82). New York: Routledge.

Harding, S. G. (1998). *Is science multicultural?: Postcolonialisms, feminisms, and epistemologies.* Bloomington: Indiana University Press.

Harding, S. G. (Ed.). (2004). *The feminist standpoint theory reader: Intellectual and political controversies.* New York: Routledge.

Hartsock, N. (1998). *The feminist standpoint revisited and other essays.* Colorado: Westview Press.

Heise, D. (1991). Event structure analysis: A qualitative model of quantitative research. In N. Fielding & R. Lee (Eds.), *Using computers in qualitative research* (pp. 136–163). London: Sage.

Heise, D., & Lewis, E. (1988). *Introduction to ETHNO.* Raleigh, NC: National Collegiate Software Clearinghouse.

Hesse-Biber, S. N. (1995). Unleashing Frankenstein's monster: The use of computers in qualitative research. *Studies in Qualitative Methodology, 5*, 25–41.

Hesse-Biber, S. N. (1996). *Am I thin enough yet?: The cult of thinness and the commercialization of identity.* New York: Oxford University Press.

Hesse-Biber, S. N. (2007). *The cult of thinness.* New York: Oxford University Press.

Hesse-Biber, S. N., & Carter, G. L. (2004). Linking qualitative and quantitative analysis: The example of family socialization and eating disorders. In G. L. Carter (Ed.), *Empirical approaches to sociology: A collection of classic and contemporary readings* (4th ed., pp. 83–97). Boston: Pearson/Allyn & Bacon.

Hesse-Biber, S. N., & Carter, G. L. (2005). *Working women in America: Split dreams* (2nd ed.). New York: Oxford University Press.

Hesse-Biber, S. N., & Crofts, C. (2008). User-centered perspective on qualitative data analysis software: Emergent technologies and future trends. In S. N. Hesse-Biber & P. Leavy (Eds.), *Handbook of emergent methods* (pp. 655–674). New York: Guilford Press.

Hesse-Biber, S. N., & Dupuis, P. (1995). Hypothesis testing in computer-aided qualitative data analysis. In U. Kelle (Ed.), *Computer-aided qualitative data analysis* (pp. 129–135). Newbury Park, CA: Sage.

Hesse-Biber, S. N., Dupuis, P., & Kinder, T. S. (1991). HyperRESEARCH: A computer program for the analysis of qualitative data with an emphasis on hypothesis testing and multimedia analysis. *Qualitative Sociology, 14,* 289–306.

Hesse-Biber, S. N., & Leavy, P. (2006a). Analysis and interpretation of qualitative data. In *The practice of qualitative research* (pp. 343–374). Thousand Oaks, CA: Sage.

Hesse-Biber, S. N., & Leavy, P. (Eds.). (2006b). *Emergent methods in social research.* Thousand Oaks, CA: Sage.

Hesse-Biber, S. N., & Leavy, P. (2006c). The ethics of social research. *The practice of qualitative research* (pp. 83–116). Thousand Oaks, CA: Sage.

Hesse-Biber, S. N., & Leavy, P. (2006d). Introduction. In S. N. Hesse-Biber & P. Leavy (Eds.), *Emergent methods in social research* (pp. ix–xxxii). Thousand Oaks, CA: Sage.

Hesse-Biber, S. N., & Leavy, P. (2006e). *The practice of qualitative research.* Thousand Oaks, CA: Sage.

Hesse-Biber, S. N., & Leavy, P. (2006f). The research process. In *The practice of qualitative research* (pp. 45–82). Thousand Oaks, CA: Sage.

Hesse-Biber, S. N., & Yaiser, M. L. (Eds.). (2004). *Feminist perspectives on social research.* New York: Oxford University Press.

Higginbotham, E. (1992, Winter). African-American women's history and the metalanguage of race. *Signs, 17*(2), 251–274.

Hodge, M. J. (2006). The fourth amendment and privacy issues on the "new" Internet: Facebook.com and Myspace.com. *Southern Illinois University Law Journal, 31,* 95–122.

hooks, b. (1989). *Talking back: Thinking feminist, thinking black.* Boston: South End Press.

hooks, b. (1990). *Yearning: Race, gender, and cultural politics.* Boston: South End Press.

hooks, b. (1992). *Black looks: Race and representation.* Boston: South End Press.

Howe, K. R. (2003). *Closing methodological divides: Toward democratic educational research.* Dordrecht, The Netherlands: Kluwer.

Howe, K. R. (2004). A critique of experimentalism. *Qualitative Inquiry, 10*(1), 42–61.

*ICARP II: Science plan 11. Arctic science in the public interest.* (2005). Retrieved June 20,

2008, from *arcticportal.org/uploads/aK/jI/aKjILkWDNnY50dJ8IAP8dw/ICARP_II_Science_Plan_11.pdf.*

Jackson, L. (1998). The influence of both race and gender on the experiences of African American college women. *Review of Higher Education, 21*(4), 359–375.

Jackson, P. T. (2006, August–September). *A statistician strikes out: In defense of genuine methodological diversity.* Paper presented at the meeting of the American Political Science Association, Philadelphia.

Jenkins, J. E. (2001). Rural adolescent perceptions of alcohol and other drug resistance. *Child Study Journal, 31*(4), 211–224.

Jick, T. D. (1979). Mixing qualitative and quantitative methods: Triangulation in action. *Administrative Science Quarterly, 24*(4), 602–611.

Johnson, R. B., & Onwuegbuzie, A. J. (2004). Mixed methods research: A research paradigm whose time has come. *Educational Researcher, 33*(7), 14–26.

Jovic, E., Wallace, J. E., & Lemaire, J. (2006). The generation and gender shifts in medicine: An exploratory survey of internal medicine physicians. *BMC Health Services Research, 6*(55).

Kantor, J. (2007, January 8). As obesity fight hits cafeteria, many fear a note from school. *The New York Times*, pp. A1, A14.

Kirby, K., Moran, A., Guerin, S., & MacIntyre, T. (2008, May). *Doping in sport: Knowledge, attitudes and psychological correlates.* Paper presented at the Annual Conference of British Psychological Society, Royal Dublin Society, Dublin.

Klein, J. T. (1990). *Interdisciplinarity: History, theory, and practice.* Detroit, MI: Wayne State University Press.

Kushner, S. (2002). I'll take mine neat: Multiple methods but a single methodology. *Evaluation, 8*(2), 249–258.

Kvale, S. (1996). *Interviews: An introduction to qualitative research interviewing.* Thousand Oaks, CA: Sage.

Le Play, F. (1855). *European workers.* Tours, France: Alfred Mame.

Lincoln, Y. S., & Guba, E. G. (1985). *Naturalistic inquiry.* Beverly Hills, CA: Sage.

Locke, L. F., Spirduso, W. W., & Silverman, S. J. (2007). *Proposals that work: A guide for planning dissertations and grant proposals.* Thousand Oaks, CA: Sage.

Lyotard, J. (1984). *The postmodern condition: A report on knowledge* (G. Bennington & B. Massumi, Trans.), Minneapolis, MN: University of Minnesota Press.

Mactavish, J. B., & Schleien, S. J. (2004). Re-injecting spontaneity and balance in family life: Parents' perspectives on recreation in families that include children with developmental disability. *Journal of Intellectual Disability Research, 48*(2), 123–141.

Mandela, N. (1993, March 27). *Keynote address by Nelson Mandela, President of the African National Congress, to the conference of the Broad Patriotic Front.* Retrieved June 19, 2008, from *www.anc.org.za/ancdocs/history/mandela/1993/sp930327.html.*

Maxwell, J. A. (1992). Understanding and validity in qualitative research. *Harvard Eduational Review, 62*(3), 279–300.

Mertens, D. (2005). *Research and evaluation in education and psychology: Integrating diversity with quantitative, qualitative, and mixed methods.* Thousand Oaks, CA: Sage.

Miles, M., & Huberman, M. (1994). *Qualitative data analysis: An expanded sourcebook* (2nd ed.). Thousand Oaks, CA: Sage.

Miller, S. J., & Fredericks, M. (2006). Mixed methods and evaluation research: Trends and issues. *Qualitative Health Research, 16*(4), 567–579.

Miner-Rubino, K., & Jayaratne, T. E. (2007). Feminist survey research. In S. Hesse-Biber & P. Leavy (Eds.), *The practice of feminist research* (pp. 293–325). Thousand Oaks, CA: Sage.

Minh-ha, T. (1992). *Framer framed.* New York: Routledge.

Mohanty, C. (1988). Under Western eyes: Feminist scholarship and colonial discourses. *Feminist Review, 30,* 61–88.

Mohanty, C. (1999). Women workers and capitalist scripts: Ideologies of domination, common interests, and the politics of solidarity. In S. N. Hesse-Biber, C. Gilmartin, & R. Lydenberg (Eds.), *Feminist approaches to theory and methodology* (pp. 362–388). New York: Oxford University Press.

Moreno, M., Fost, N., & Christakis, D. (2008). Research ethics in the MySpace era. *Pediatrics, 121,* 157–161.

Morgan, D. (1998). Practical strategies for combining qualitative and quantitative methods: Applications to health research. *Qualitative Health Journal, 8*(3), 362–376.

Morse, J. M. (1995). The significance of saturation. *Qualitative Health Research, 5,* 147–149.

Morse, J. M. (2003). Principles of mixed methods and multimethod research design. In A. Tashakkori & C. Teddlie (Eds.), *Handbook of mixed methods in social and behavioral research* (pp. 189–208). Thousand Oaks, CA: Sage.

Morse, J. M. (2006). The politics of developing research methods. *Qualitative Health Research, 16*(3), 3–4.

Nicholson, P. (2004). Taking quality seriously: The case for qualitative feminist psychology in the context of quantitative clinical research on postnatal depression. In Z. Todd, B. Nerlich, S. McDeown, & D. D. Clarke (Eds.), *Mixing methods in psychology: The integration of qualitative and quantitative methods in theory and practice* (pp. 201–224). New York: Psychology Press.

Nickel, B., Berger, M., Schmidt, P., & Plies, K. (1995). Qualitative sampling in a multi-method study: Practical problems of method triangulation in sexual behavior research. *Quality and Quantity, 29*(3), 223–240.

Nielsen, J. M. (Ed.). (1990). *Feminist research methods: Exemplary readings in the social sciences.* Boulder, CO: Westview Press.

Nightingale, A. (2003). A feminist in the forest: Situated knowledges and mixing methods in natural resource management. *ACME: An International E-Journal for Critical Geographers, 2*(1), 77–90.

Nightingale, A. (2006a). The nature of gender: Work, gender, and environment. *Environment and Planning D: Society and Space, 24*(2), 165–185.

Nightingale, A. (2006b). *A forest community or community forestry? Beliefs, meanings and nature in north-western Nepal* (Institute of Geography Online Paper Series, GEO-026). Available at *www.era.lib.ed.ac.uk/bitstream/1842/1436/1/anightingale003.pdf.*

O'Loughlin, J., Ó Tuathail, G., & Kolossov, V. (2004a). A "risky westward turn"? Putin's 9-11 script and ordinary Russians. *Europe–Asia Studies, 56*(1), 3–34.

O'Loughlin, J., Ó Tuathail, G., & Kolossov, V. (2004b). Russian geopolitical storylines and public opinion in the wake of 9-11: A critical geopolitical analysis and national survey. *Communist and Post-Communist Studies, 37,* 281–318.

Onwuegbuzie, A. J., & Collins, K. M. T. (2007). A typology of mixed methods sampling designs in social science research. *The Qualitative Report, 12*(2), 281–316. Available at *www.nova.edu/ssss/QR/QR12-2/onwuegbuzie2.pdf.*

Onwuegbuzie, A. J., & Johnson, R. B. (2006). The validity issue in mixed research. *Research in the Schools, 13*(1), 48–63.

Onwuegbuzie, A. J., & Leech, N. L. (2006). Linking research questions to mixed methods data analysis procedures. *Qualitative Report, 11*(3), 474–498.

Oral History Project Team. (2007). The oral history of evaluation: Part 5. An interview with Michael Quinn Patton. *American Journal of Evaluation, 28*, 102–114.

Parker, L. (1992). *Discourse dynamics: Critical analysis for social and individual psychology.* London: Routledge.

Patton, M. Q. (1999). *Grand Canyon celebration: A father–son journey of discovery.* Amherst, NY: Prometheus Books.

Patton, M. Q. (2002). *Qualitative research and evaluation methods* (3rd ed.). Thousand Oaks, CA: Sage.

Platt, J. (1996). *A history of sociological research methods in America, 1920–1960.* Cambridge, UK: Cambridge University Press.

Pope, H., Phillips, K., & Olivardi, R. (2000). *The Adonis complex: The secret crisis of male body obsession.* New York: Simon & Schuster.

Pumping up your body image. (2002, April–May). *Current Health, 2.*

Ragin, C. C. (2000). *Fuzzy-set social science.* Chicago, IL: University of Chicago Press.

Reay, D. (1998). *Class work: Mothers' involvement in their children's schooling.* London: University College Press.

Reed, M. G. (2003a). Marginality and gender at work in forestry communities in British Columbia, Canada. *Journal of Rural Studies, 19*, 373–389.

Reed, M. G. (2003b). *Taking stands: Gender and the sustainability of rural communities.* Vancouver, British Columbia, Canada: University of British Columbia Press.

Reinharz, S. (1992). *Feminist methods in social research.* New York: Oxford University Press.

Richardson, L. (1994). Writing a method of inquiry. In N. K. Denzin & F. S. Lincoln (Eds.), *Handbook of qualitative research* (pp. 516–529). Thousand Oaks, CA: Sage.

Roberts, H. (Ed.). (1981). *Doing feminist research.* London: Routledge.

Rosenau, P. M. (1992). *Post-modernism and the social sciences: Insights, inroads, and intrusions.* Princeton, NJ: Princeton University Press.

Rowntree, B. S. (1901). *Poverty: A study of town life.* London: Macmillan.

Sandelowski, M. (2000a). Combining qualitative and quantitative sampling, data collection, and analysis techniques in mixed-method studies. *Research in Nursing and Health, 23*(3), 246–255.

Sandelowski, M. (2000b). Focus on research methods: Whatever happened to qualitative description? *Research in Nursing and Health, 23*, 334–340.

Sandelowski, M., Volis, C. I., & Knafl, G. (2009). On quantizing. *Journal of Mixed Methods Research, 3*(3), 208–222.

Sieber, S. D. (1973). The integration of fieldwork and survey methods. *American Journal of Sociology, 78*(6), 1335–1359.

Simons, L. (2007). Moving from collision to integration: Reflecting on the experience of mixed methods. *Journal of Research in Nursing, 12*(1), 73–83.

Smith, D. E. (1987a). Women's perspective as a radical critique of sociology. *Sociological Inquiry, 44*, 7–13.

Smith, D. E. (1987b). *The everyday world as problematic: A feminist sociology.* Boston: Northeastern University Press.

Spivak, G. C. (1994). Can the subaltern speak? In P. Williams & L. Chrismen (Eds.), *Colonial discourse and postcolonial theory: A reader* (pp. 66–111). New York: Columbia University Press.

Sprague, J., & Zimmerman, M. K. (2004). Overcoming dualisms: A feminist agenda for sociological methodology. In S. N. Hesse-Biber & P. Leavy (Eds.), *Approaches to qualitative research: A reader on theory and practice* (pp. 39–61). New York: Oxford University Press.

Tashakkori, A., & Teddlie, C. (Eds.). (1998). *Mixed methodology: Combining qualitative and quantitative approaches.* Thousand Oaks, CA: Sage.

Tashakkori, A., & Teddlie, C. (Eds.). (2003). *Handbook of mixed methods in social and behavioral research.* Thousand Oaks, CA: Sage.

Teddlie, C., & Tashakkori, A. (2008). *Foundations of mixed methods research: Integrating quantitative and qualitative approaches in the behavioral and social sciences.* Thousand Oaks, CA: Sage.

Tesch, R. (1990). *Qualitative research: Analysis types and software tools.* New York: Falmer Press.

Thomas, C. (2000). *Straight with a twist: Queer theory and the subject of heterosexuality.* Champaign: University of Illinois Press.

Tolman, D. L., & Szalacha, L. A. (1999). Dimensions of desire: Bridging qualitative and quantitative methods in a study of female adolescent sexuality. *Psychology of Women Quarterly, 23*, 7–39.

Wang, Y., & Beydouns, M. A. (2007). The obesity epidemic in the United States: Gender, age, socioeconomic, racial/ethnic, and geographic characteristics. A systematic review and meta-regression analysis. *Epidemiologic Reviews, 29*(1), 6–28.

Weber, L. (1998). A conceptual framework for understanding race, class, gender, and sexuality. *Psychology of Women Quarterly, 22*, 13–32.

Weitzman, E. A., & Miles, M. B. (1995). *Computer programs for qualitative data analysis.* Thousand Oaks, CA: Sage.

Westhues, A., Ochocka, J., Jacobson, N., Simich, L., Maiter, S., Janzen, R., et al. (2008). Developing theory from complexity: Reflections on a collaborative mixed methods participatory action research study. *Qualitative Health Research, 18*(5), 701–717.

Weston, D., & Rofel, L. (1984). Sexuality, class, and conflict in a lesbian workplace. *Signs, 9*(4), 623–646.

Wing, A. K. (Ed.). (2000). *Global critical race feminism: An international reader.* New York: New York University Press.

Winters, C. (2007, September). The second annual *Ladies' Home Journal* health breakthrough awards. Available at *www.lhj.com/lhj/printableStory.jhtml;jsessionid=AUIPCAKJZGTPBQFIBQNSCAQ?storyid=/templatedata/lhj/story/data/1186606396633.xml&catref=bcat66.*

Yauch, C. A., & Steudel, H. J. (2003). Complementary use of qualitative and quantitative cultural assessment methods. *Organizational Research Methods, 6*(4), 465–481.

# Author Index

# Subject Index

"*f*" following a page number indicates a figure;
"*t*" following a page number indicates a table;
page numbers in bold indicate glossary terms.

# About the Author

Sharlene Nagy Hesse-Biber, PhD, is Professor of Sociology and Director of Women's Studies at Boston College in Chestnut Hill, Massachusetts. She is also the founder and former Executive Director of the National Association for Women in Catholic Higher Education. Dr. Hesse-Biber has published widely on the impact of sociocultural factors on women's body image, including the books *Am I Thin Enough Yet?: The Cult of Thinness and the Commercialization of Identity* (1996), which was selected as one of *Choice* magazine's best academic books for 1996, and *The Cult of Thinness* (2007). She is coauthor of *Working Women in America: Split Dreams* (2005) and *The Practice of Qualitative Research* (2006); coeditor of *Approaches to Qualitative Research: A Reader on Theory and Practice* (2004), *Emergent Methods in Social Research* (2006), and *Handbook of Emergent Methods* (2008); and editor of *Handbook of Feminist Research: Theory and Praxis* (2007), which was selected as one of the Critics Choice Award winners by the American Educational Studies Association and as one of *Choice* magazine's outstanding academic titles for 2007. She is also a contributor to the *Handbook of Grounded Theory* (2008) and editor of the forthcoming book *Handbook of Emergent Technologies in Social Research*. Dr. Hesse-Biber is codeveloper of the software program HyperRESEARCH, a computer-assisted program for analyzing qualitative data, and the new transcription tool HyperTRANSCRIBE (*www.researchware.com*).

# About the Contributing Author

**Chris Kelly,** a contributor to Chapter 6, "Postmodernist Approaches to Mixed Methods Research," is a PhD student in the Department of Sociology at Boston College. His academic interests include the sociology of knowledge, qualitative methods, discourse analysis, queer and post-colonial studies, Islam, and spirituality. His past work has addressed knowledge in social movement organizations, and he has also done work examining queer issues in Islam and Muslim communities, which will likely be the focus of his dissertation.

# About the Researchers Interviewed

**Stephen P. Borgatti, PhD,** is Chellgren Endowed Chair and Professor in the Department of Management, Gatton College of Business and Economics, University of Kentucky. He taught at the University of California, Riverside, the University of South Carolina, and the Carroll School of Management at Boston College before coming to the University of Kentucky in 2007. His research focuses on social networks of all kinds, group culture, and knowledge management (which he regards as the intersection of networks and culture). Recent publications include "A Graph-theoretic Perspective on Centrality" (*Social Networks*), "The Network Paradigm in Organizational Research: A Review and Typology" (*Journal of Management*), and the KeyPlayer program (National Academies Press).

**Julianne Cheek, PhD,** is Professor at the Institute of Nursing and Health Sciences at the University of Oslo and also Professor in the School of Health Sciences at the University of South Australia. She is widely published, including her book *Postmodern and Poststructural Approaches to Nursing Research* (2000). Dr. Cheek is an associate editor of *Qualitative Health Research* and sits on the editorial boards of a number of journals with an interest in qualitative methods. Her three major interests are the development of methodological understandings pertaining to qualitative research, with an emphasis on funded research; research in the substantive area of care of the older person; and the application of Foucauldian and postmodern perspectives to health care.

**David A. Karp, PhD,** is Professor of Sociology at Boston College. His publications include *The Burden of Sympathy: How Families Cope with Mental Illness* (2002); *Speaking of Sadness: Depression, Disconnection, and the Meanings of Illness* (1997); *Being Urban: A Sociology of City Life* (1994); *Sociology in Everyday Life* (1993); *Experiencing the Life Cycle: A Social Psychology of Aging* (1993); and *The Research Craft: An Introduction to Social Research Methods* (1992).

**Andrea Nightingale, PhD,** is Lecturer in Geography at the University of Edinburgh, as well as Director of Studies (MA Geography) and Director of Studies (BSc Geography). She specializes in working at the social–natural science interface. Dr. Nightingale's present research focuses on the management of common property resources to integrate an analysis of the social politics of resource use with an evaluation of ecological change. Her research interests build from her background in ecological science, political economy, and feminist theory to thinking through questions of natural resource management; taking seriously critiques of "nature"; the need to incorporate ecology into a social-political analysis; and close engagement with questions of power, inequalities, and governance.